Maternity
Leave

Praeclarus Press, LLC
2504 Sweetgum Lane
Amarillo, Texas 79124 USA
806-367-9950
www.PraeclarusPress.com

DISCLAIMER
The information contained in this publication is advisory only and is not intended to replace sound clinical judgment or individualized patient care. The author disclaims all warranties, whether expressed or implied, including any warranty as the quality, accuracy, safety, or suitability of this information for any particular purpose.

ISBN: 9781939807434

Cover Design: Ken Tackett
Illustrations: Ken Tackett
Copy Editing: Chris Tackett
Acquisition & Development: Kathleen Kendall-Tackett
Layout & Design: Cornelia Georgiana Murariu
Operations: Scott Sherwood

Maternity Leave

A New Mother's Guide to the First Six Weeks Postpartum

Cheryl R. Zauderer, PhD, CNM, NPP, IBCLC

Praeclarus Press, LLC

www.PraeclarusPress.com

Contents

Foreword

Wendy N. Davis, PhD

How can I be so happy yet so utterly exhausted at the same time?

I keep on forgetting things.

What has happened to my body?

Am I supposed to bond or attach with my baby right away?

How can dad attach?

I love my baby— how can I be feeling depressed?

When will I feel like having sex again?

What happened to my social life?

I didn't know how badly I was feeling, until I started to feel good again.

When I was a vulnerable new mother, I asked myself all these questions echoed in this resourceful book by Dr Cheryl Zauderer. I know, without doubt, that I would have been so encouraged and informed had I found this guide. I survived, managed to find information. and recovered to become an advocate and expert in perinatal mental health and recovery myself. When I was that new mom, I collected information in bits and pieces from some seminal books and a few providers, but I ask myself: what if I had one book, perfectly readable as this one, to read while caring for my baby? And more, what if I had this amazing book that reminded me that I could (and should) care for myself right alongside caring for my baby? It took me two babies, and a recovery from a postpartum mood disorder, to understand the important preventive factor of that self-care. Here in this book Cheryl lays it out with simplicity and compassion.

In this unique guide, Cheryl Zauderer speaks to us with the most potent mixture of reassurance and research. This essential book draws on her extensive knowledge and experience, enhanced by the fact that she is not only an expert clinician and researcher, but is also a mother and astute listener. Reading her book, we feel that we are in good hands, and imagine the comfort and security that her clients and babies must feel. I think about all those initials behind her name and realize we are receiving knowledge gleaned from so many hours of real life and scholarly immersion: Lactation Consultant; Psychiatric Nurse Practitioner; Certified Nurse Midwife; Doctor of Psychology; Assistant Professor at the Department of Nursing at the New York Institute of Technology.

As well as the importance of her job as a mother, the additional credential Cheryl has with no post-name initials, is that she has been a dedicated volunteer Coordinator for Postpartum Support International since 2009, helping and finding resources for women and families in her own community. In my work as a psychotherapist and Executive Director of Postpartum Support International (PSI), this is exactly the kind of book we look for: one that I can recommend to families with security that they will find both compassionate reassurance and solid information, backed by references and resources, for families.

New mothers, families, and their providers need the information and wisdom in this book. In our modern world we have an increasing technological ability to monitor and measure our births and babies, but we have lost the essential transmission of knowledge and information to teach parents how to support their bodies, emotional life, and relationships during the postpartum period and beyond. This book provides what parents need to know about how to listen to their own needs and instincts, replenish after birth, and nurture themselves so they can nurture their babies. *Maternity Leave* is a needed contribution to the world of childbirth and postpartum recovery, providing thorough and non-judgmental information about the early days, childbirth recovery including cesarean birth, breast and bottle feeding, nutrition, sexuality, bonding, work-family balance, postpartum emotional recovery, and resources.

Cheryl writes in the last chapter, *"The first 6 weeks after childbirth is all about protecting and nurturing your newborn. Your baby needs you now more than she ever will again. The first 6 weeks are difficult, and you may feel isolated and trapped. There is a fine line between embracing motherhood, and nourishing yourself as an individual. It's very hard, but it's worth it."*

I add my enthusiastic agreement and appreciation for this book, and am grateful for the guidance Maternity Leave gives to parents during this vulnerable and powerful time in their lives.

Wendy Newhouse Davis, PhD
Executive Director, Postpartum Support International
www.postpartum.net
Counseling & Consultation
Portland Oregon

Acknowledgements

They say that bringing home a new baby is the most exciting and rewarding experience a new mother and her partner will encounter. My inspiration for writing this book came from wanting to help new mothers receive the education and support they need during first six weeks postpartum so that they can have an easier transition into their new role as a mother.

I wish to personally thank the following people for their contributions to my vision and in helping me to create this book:

Thank you to Dr. Kathleen Kendall-Tackett, my publisher and editor, for believing in me, and my first book, and for her guidance, support, and expertise.

Thank you to Dr. Leslie Nicoll, my editor, who kept me on my toes and helped me to develop as a writer. Thank you Carolyn Luber, and Shelly Talmud, my proofreaders, whose meticulous attention to details helped to make this project as accurate and flawless as possible.

Thank you to all of the new mothers I have cared for over the years for trusting me and for sharing with me the most intimate event in your lives.

I am grateful for my own mother, Deany Ehrenreich, for coming to stay with me for two weeks after each of my four children were born. Her support and presence helped to give me the time and space to heal emotionally and physically from each of my births.

I am especially grateful to my four children, Michael, Keith, Stephanie, and Jordan, who gave me the gift of motherhood and continuously make me proud of who they are.

I am indebted to my wonderful husband, Jeff, who has given me his unrelenting support throughout this project, and has supported and encouraged me throughout my entire career.

Introduction
Your Journey into Motherhood

Embracing Motherhood

Giving life to another human being is the most spiritual and wonderful experience that a woman will ever encounter. It is a life-changing event, and in many cultures, it is looked upon as a miracle and a blessing. As a new mother, you will experience many reactions to the adjustment of your body, your postpartum recovery, and your new role. You will discover how your new role will change your life. Some new mothers feel strong and confident immediately after giving birth, but for others, this takes a little more time. You may feel yourself fighting your own insecurities as you try and create your own identity as a mother.

For many women, having a baby is the highlight of their lives. You may not remember the details of a movie or a show, or your last vacation. You may not remember what you ate for dinner or breakfast, where you were last Thanksgiving, or what you did for your anniversary. But you will probably remember all the details of your child's birth: your labor and delivery nurses, how you felt during labor, what you experienced after seeing your newborn for the first time, and the details of when you brought your newborn home.

Coming home with a new baby is not easy. Don't forget that it took you nine months to grow your baby, but only hours to birth her. You have been transformed into being a mother along with new roles that are challenging, no matter how wonderful they are. If you already have children, you may be wondering how you will do this all over again. In the first few weeks postpartum, you may be on an emotional roller coaster. You may doubt yourself in your ability to care for this new person. Instruction booklets are given out every time you buy a new car or an appliance, but a newborn does not come with instructions.

How can I be so happy yet so utterly exhausted at the same time?

On a physical level you may be sore, tired, and generally uncomfortable. Together with all the physical discomforts and challenges that you may be experiencing, your ability to focus on the simplest things can be compromised. Your whole life has changed. Your body, your relationship with your partner, your newborn, and your home may all be in a state of disarray. You may still be in a small one-bedroom apartment and feel cramped with all your new baby paraphernalia lying around. You may be in the process of moving to a larger place, or may have already moved. You may have purchased a home in the suburbs away from the city where you lived as a couple or a single woman. You may feel a bit isolated and lonely, or preoccupied with trying to get ready to return to work. You are adapting to many changes and you need support at this time in your life.

What happened to my social life?

You may be one of the first of your friends who has had a baby, and you may possibly feel a bit distanced from them right now. They may not understand how you are feeling and why your relationship with them has changed. Eventually, they will see the joy you are experiencing and accept you as a new mother. Ask them for help, get them involved with caring for your newborn, and include them in your life as much as possible. Eventually they will gain a new respect for you and what you are doing. You may even inspire them to venture into motherhood themselves!

Learning Your Newborn

As a new mother, you may be showered with advice and suggestions about how to raise your newborn, and take care of your house and home. It is important to listen to your own intuition and instinct. This is a sensitive time, the first six-to-eight weeks after birth. You and your baby have to learn each other. You have a heightened sensitivity in the early postpartum period making you very responsive to the needs of your newborn. You can certainly take cues and advice from others, but nothing is as good as your own intuition. Listen to your body and listen to your inner voice when it comes to caring for yourself and your newborn. Your emotions as well as your instincts will be very strong at this time in your life. No one knows your newborn as well as you do, and no one will take care of her the way you will.

Trust Your Own Instincts

No matter how well you mother your newborn, you may still experience a feeling of guilt for not being better at it. You may compare yourself to other mothers who seem to have it more together or are coping with it better than you are. The truth is, you don't always know what is going on in someone else's home. They may have more help, or other areas in their lives can be suffering, and they may be just making a good appearance. Don't give in to these messages and don't feel guilty for not doing it all.

Being a woman, especially a new mother in modern times, is challenging. You are learning to cope with unforeseen circumstances in life, and new motherhood. As wonderful as new motherhood is, it is a huge change and challenge, with a multitude of new emotions and feelings that come along with it. On an emotional level, you may be feeling a combination of sheer bliss, excitement, and euphoria, along with a sense of panic and exhaustion. You are now realizing that you have become transformed into a mother in a matter of hours, with a tremendous amount of responsibility, and you wonder if you will be able to adjust and handle it all. With pregnancy hormones plummeting, and breastfeeding hormones rising, your moods and emotions are extremely fragile and should be handled with loving care. There has never been a time in your life when you have had this many changes to your body and your mind.

Balance

It's all about balance! You can't expect to take care of others without taking care of yourself first. When you're on an airplane, the flight attendant will tell you to put the oxygen mask on yourself before you put it on your child or anyone else. Similarly, you can't care for your newborn if you are rundown. You need to take care of yourself and your body. During the first six weeks postpartum, you should be doing nothing but eating, sleeping, and feeding your baby. You should be practicing skin-to-skin contact with your newborn as much as possible (see Chapter 3 Post-Baby Breastfeeding). You may also begin to do some mild exercise if your health care provider gives you the okay.

This is a challenging time, but it can also be rewarding. I want to guide you through it and help you get the care and support you need.

Chapter 1
Momnesia:
The Post-Baby Brain

"I keep on forgetting things."
"I don't feel as 'with it' as I used to feel."
"I am constantly walking into a room and
forgetting what I went in there for."
"I feel as though I am in a mental fog."

"Momnesia," "Mommy Brain," or "Pregnancy Brain" are terms that are often used to describe a new mother who does not feel as "sharp" as she did prior to her pregnancy. It's a type of amnesia that you, as a new mother, may experience after birth (Brizendine, 2006; Kim, Leckman, Mayes, Feldman, Wang, & Swain, 2010). You may have occasional memory lapses and moments of forgetfulness. You may forget even the simplest things and can't seem to remember something from one minute to the next. You may be experiencing confusion, and are having a difficult time making even the smallest decisions. Don't despair! There is a scientific cause for this, and it is an actual type of memory syndrome. You are in a right brain state at the moment, and this is exactly where you need to be at this time in order to bond and attach to your newborn.

Your Brain Archetype

Your body has gone through a large number of adjustments, but the changes to your brain are your biggest challenge. Motherhood changes you in so many ways. It transforms the way you think and feel about almost everything. Your brain itself also changes (Kim et al., 2010).

As we will see, these changes to your thinking and feeling can be nature's way of making sure our species continues to evolve.

How Do These Changes Occur?

Giving birth and producing another life is a rite of passage. It is your personal journey into motherhood. It took nine months to develop and produce your new little individual, and it will take time for you to develop and evolve as a mother. Although your natural instincts about parenting will set in, you still have a lot of adjusting to do. Momnesia is the result of biological and hormonal changes that you have just experienced during pregnancy and childbirth, and are continuing to experience now during your postpartum period (Brunton, Russell, & Hirst, 2014; Kim et al., 2010). Other causes of momnesia can be general fatigue and discomfort from the challenges of childbirth. Having close contact with your newborn can also cause momnesia. As a result of this intense physical contact, your emotions will intensify making you and your newborn emotionally and physically sensitive to each other.

The Love Hormone

Did you know that there is such a thing as a Love Hormone? There are many terms used to describe the hormone that has changed your life as a new mother. It is the bonding hormone, the "falling in love" hormone, the cuddle chemical, the trust hormone, and the healing hormone. This hormone is known as *oxytocin* (Bartz, Zaki, Bolger, & Ochsner, 2011; Fletcher, Simpson, Campbell, & Overall, 2015; Uvnas-Moberg, 2003).

What is Oxytocin?

Oxytocin is a hormone that is produced by the hypothalamus (part of the brain that creates hormones), and released from the posterior pituitary (part of the brain that stores and releases these hormones into the circulation). This hormone has been studied extensively (Cong, Ludington-Hoe, Hussain, Cusson, Walsh, Vazquez et al., 2015; Fletcher et al., 2014). Oxytocin not only plays a role in pregnancy and the postpartum period, but also many other factors unrelated to pregnancy. For the most part, oxytocin is responsible for the initiation of labor contractions and the release of milk during breastfeeding.

Oxytocin is believed to be responsible for other behaviors such as attachment, romance, lust, increased libido, and sexual satisfaction; it also promotes wound healing and reduces inflammation. Additionally, oxytocin has been found to increase trust and reduce fear. In the breast-feeding mother, oxytocin is released in response to your newborn's sucking, and initiates the milk-ejection reflex, also known as the letdown reflex. Letdown causes contractions and helps bring the milk out of the milk ducts, making it available to the newborn. Oxytocin will also help your uterus to contract, and return to its normal size, helping to control your postpartum bleeding (Pillitteri, 2014; Ricci, Kyle, & Carman, 2013). These contractions will trigger some cramping during and after you breastfeed your newborn.

Oxytocin will dilate your blood vessels, increasing blood flow throughout your body. This increase in blood flow will raise your skin temperature and produce a calming effect on you, which in turn, will produce a calming effect on your newborn. Oxytocin is released during "skin-to-skin" contact with your newborn. Many studies have shown that mothers and babies thrive when they are in close contact with each other—your newborn's bare skin against your bare skin. According to Colson (2005), skin-to-skin contact is not always required for breastfeeding and bonding. Some mothers may not want to undress their newborns every time they feed, or undress themselves. New mothers and babies can receive these same effects when both are lightly clothed, or the newborn is lightly swaddled. Holding your newborn close and cuddling with her will release oxytocin and enhance your bonding experience.

How Do I apply Skin-to-Skin Contact?

Your newborn's chest should be placed against your bare chest, between your breasts. Your newborn baby should be naked except for a diaper and a hat, and wrapped under blankets or a robe together with you.

Skin-to-skin contact has gained much popularity in hospital settings immediately after birth, and its continuation is encouraged once the mother and newborn are discharged home for as long as you both wish. With skin-to-skin contact, breastfeeding becomes easier for your newborn, and his or her temperature remains stable. Oxytocin will help you learn your newborn's cues, produce more milk, and help calm you and your newborn (Skin-to-skin contact will be discussed in more detail in Chapters 4 and 5).

If you are breastfeeding, oxytocin will also be released as soon as your newborn grabs a hold of your breast, attaches to the nipple, and continues to be released through your newborn's suckling (Colson, 2005; Cong et al., 2015; Rice-Simpson & Creehan, 2014). Your newborn will become familiar with your odor and warmth. Oxytocin will help your newborn associate these familiar cues with breastfeeding. This will help your newborn to continue to feed, while gaining the benefits of skin-to-skin contact.

If you are not breastfeeding, oxytocin can still be released through skin-to-skin contact, and you can certainly initiate this bonding approach with your newborn. As a bottle-feeding mom, you and your newborn can achieve many of the benefits associated with oxytocin release, such as a feeling of calm, a decrease in stress, and an increase in bonding and social attachment. Oxytocin also creates an anti-stress effect, causing sedation and a feeling of calm, which can cause you to feel relaxed and even slightly unfocused.

Science of Love

All of these hormonal changes may have an effect on the way you think and feel, as you become more and more preoccupied with your newborn. You have developed an increased awareness into your newborn and his needs. In order for your newborn's needs to be met, it is essential to have complete maternal preoccupation. There are certain parts of your brain that are responsible for focusing and concentrating that are now preoccupied with being responsible for caring for your newborn. The hormones that are released during breastfeeding or skin-to-skin contact can cause your brain to form new connections. They take over any new mother's brain, whether you are career driven or have the desire to be a stay-at-home mom, changing the way you think, feel, and what you perceive as important. The hormonal and metabolic changes that occur in your body during pregnancy and postpartum stimulate your brain to reassure you, as a new mother, to have the confidence to care for your newborn when he arrives (Brunton et al., 2014).

Mother Love

Loving your newborn can cause you to feel mentally disorganized and unfocused, but you will become entranced with cuddling your newborn and actually feel withdrawal when you are separated. You will develop a passion and determination to care for and shelter your newborn in a way you never felt before. Your brain has changed, along with your devotion and loyalty, and a new sense of protectiveness comes over you. Most animals become extremely hypervigilant and protective over their litters. They will even reject an offspring from a different litter because they don't recognize or associate with its scent. In a similar way, as you inhale your newborn's scent, see and hear him, and touch the very soft newborn skin, you become absorbed into an almost dream-like state with loving feelings for your child. The experience of the pleasant smell of your newborn's head starts a chemical reaction in your brain—his scent will be imprinted there for a long time. Other baby smells and odors, such as bodily fluids, spit up, and sweat, will also be imprinted on your brain, and you will begin to feel a wave of protectiveness when you're with your newborn. A new mother can pick out her own baby's scent and cries from other babies. Oxytocin is again stimulated by the sweet smell of your newborn's little body.

Baby Talk

A change in priorities can also cause you to become more forgetful and mentally foggy. Your brain is currently more right-brain focused, being more intuitive during this time. You are now preoccupied with taking care of your newborn and becoming comfortable with your new role as a mother. You may become overly attentive, alert about safety in the home, and concerned about germs, protecting your "nest" at all times. New mothers develop a shift in memory priority; the types of things that you remember are different from before. You may remember *everything* related to your newborn, including when he ate and was changed, how long he slept, and his daily habits. You will be more alert for changes or warning signs. These changes can also be seen in adoptive mothers. Continuing to have close physical contact with your newborn, especially skin-to-skin contact, will cause the release of oxytocin in your brain, which will maintain your new sense of momnesia.

Lifting the Fog

While there are many benefits to momnesia, it can be somewhat frustrating if you are trying to function and get some things done outside of your home. There are many steps that you can take towards improving your memory to help you better manage the first six weeks of your life with your newborn.

Mothering the New Mother

Historically, in certain cultures, extended families may have lived together. Within this network, social support was already built in, and provided by siblings, mothers, grandmothers, and great-grandmothers. If this were to occur, then by the time the new mother would have gone back into society, she would have been rested, refreshed, and her body would have been healed. She would have established her milk supply based on her newborn's needs, and become comfortable with feeding and caring for her newborn. She would have bonded with her newborn, and vice versa, and learned his or her routine. Mother and baby would be in-sync, together, as a mother-newborn dyad.

The United States is one of the few industrialized countries where postpartum supportive care for the new mother is not automatic. Postpartum disorders are much lower in some other countries. There are, however, certain cultures in the United States that do have protective social structures built into their traditions with regards to postpartum care for new mothers (Zauderer, 2009, 2012). These cultures allow for a recuperation period, where the new mother is forced to rest. Her activities are restricted and female relatives and, other mothers in the community help take care of her physical needs and help her to adjust to her life with her newborn. This help, in turn, improves her emotional needs. The new mother typically does nothing but eat, rest, and feed her newborn for a certain length of time that varies among cultures. Some cultures apply this rule for 90 days. In some cultures, the women even bathe and massage the new mother. Household help is taken care of, and if she has other children, they are taken care of as well (Semenic, Callister, & Feldman, 2004).

Learning to Accept Help

Although you may enjoy your autonomy and feel confident that you can do this all on your own, it is still a good idea to enlist some help. You will have some very good days, but also some not-so-good days. As you are healing both mentally and physically, it is a good idea to have an extra pair of hands around. You may not be accustomed to other people in your home, waiting on you, or touching your belongings. Try to let go of control so that you can focus on the important things, like healing from birth and understanding your newborn. If you are fortunate enough to have help from your partner, family, friends, or even hired help, allow them to take care of your house, do the laundry, cook a meal, and shop for you. Let someone hold a crying newborn for you so that you can take a relaxing shower without worrying. If your partner can take off from work, that will be very useful, but you may still need extra help in the home.

If you can plan ahead, you can arrange for family members or close friends who you feel comfortable with to spend at least a week or two with you. If you can't get anyone to do this, and you can afford it, you can hire someone to come to the home on a temporary basis. A postpartum doula or nanny can all take the place of a relative, as long as you don't allow them to take over and interrupt your feedings or your bonding experience with your newborn. Set limits, give clear instruction as to what their responsibilities are, and don't allow them to influence your own instinctual behaviors.

Many mothers receive care and support from a doula during labor. If you did not have the opportunity to have doula support in labor, you can certainly hire one for the postpartum period. A postpartum doula is trained in providing postpartum support to the mother and can help you with your physical needs, the needs of your newborn, and sometimes your emotional needs as well. She can offer a world of knowledge and wisdom, education, and camaraderie during your recovery phase. She can teach you some coping skills and provide invaluable support during this time.

During the postpartum period, you will need emotional and physical support, domestic help, resources, and a culture that values motherhood. Try to surround yourself with warm, supportive people and search for a good support team, and embrace them and their advice. Let them know what your needs are. Surrounding yourself with supportive loved ones is not a luxury, it is a necessity!

Sleep, Sleep, Sleep

As much as you can, whenever you can, wherever you can! A newborn can drain your energy and you will experience a lack of sleep like you never have before. If this is your first baby, you probably were used to going to sleep when you wanted to, sleeping in on weekends and holidays, and showering and grooming yourself on a regular basis. Who wouldn't expect to be able to do these things? This all changes once your newborn arrives. Now, those simple things become a luxury! Aside from your own body healing, and dealing with physical discomforts, you now have a human being who is dependent on you in every way. You need to care for this individual 24/7. That means all day long, and all night long as well. If you are lucky and have the type of newborn who will sleep in between nighttime feedings, you have half the battle won. Hopefully, all of that oxytocin combined with sheer exhaustion will enable you to fall asleep after a feeding, along with your newborn. Even in this best-case scenario, however, you will end up with broken sleep, which is something your body is not used to.

Try to nap during the day if at all possible, and sleep whenever your newborn sleeps, even if it is for a short time. Don't attempt to take care of household chores while your newborn is sleeping. If you can even get a few winks of rest or sleep during the day, you will be much better off than having a clean and organized household. It would be a good idea for you to lower your expectations of a clean house. Your home does not have to be spotless, nor does it have to be perfect—it should feel lived in and comfortable. Letting things go for now is the best thing you can do.

You may have the type of newborn who does not go back to sleep after a nighttime feeding. Your newborn may have gas and need to burp, or just continue to be fussy in general. This can cause you to be up quite a bit during the night. You may have good nights, and you may have bad nights. That feeling of sleep deprivation can make you feel almost like a zombie throughout the day. As best as you can, try to establish some form of sleep schedule. Go to sleep for the night soon after your baby does. Video screens, such as those found on computers, tablets, smart phones, and televisions can stimulate your brain and delay falling asleep. It is good sleep hygiene, just in general, to not watch TV or use electronics for at least an hour before going to bed.

You will need every bit of sleep that you can get during the first six weeks postpartum. If you are having trouble falling asleep, and you have the time and energy, try to soak in a hot bath. You can add some lavender and Epsom salts to make it more relaxing. You can light some scented candles too. Get into a routine so that you can create a regular, peaceful, and tranquil bedtime routine. As best as you can, create an environment that is conducive to sleep. Keep your bedroom dark, quiet, and comfortable. Try not to have a lot of clutter around, but have some light reading available, such as magazines or an interesting novel.

Food for Thought

A well-balanced diet will not only help you improve your memory, but will increase your energy and make you feel a whole lot stronger all around (Lim, Barnett-Lopez, & Franciso, 2004; Seetharaman, Andel, McEvoy, Aslan, Finkel, & Pedersen, 2015; Zuniga & McAuley, 2015). Don't forget who else is getting the benefits of your healthy diet—your newborn! Avoid or reduce sugar and caffeine intake. They will both give you a burst of energy at first, but then will cause a drop in both energy and focus. Caffeine and sugar can make you feel anxious and stressed, and can cause poor brain function.

Drink plenty of water. Staying hydrated is very important for you. Dehydration may cause you to have decreased memory and can also cause confusion. You need to have adequate amounts of water for positive cognitive functioning. Caffeine or alcohol can cause you to become dehydrated. Dehydration from exercise, water restriction, and excessive heat can impair cognitive function (Benefer, Corfe, Russell, Short, & Barker, 2013). Aim for the equivalent of 6 to 8 eight-ounce glasses of water every day. You can purchase a portable water bottle that can hold 32 or 64 ounces of water and keep refilling it throughout the day. Get one that can be carried around with you easily. Always sit down with a water bottle or a glass of water when you're about to breastfeed your baby. Breastfeeding does make you thirsty, which is a reminder to rehydrate.

Eating fruits and vegetables that have high water content in them can add to hydration and supply you with proper nutrients. Now is not the time to diet; this is the time to eat healthy. Always start with a good breakfast, which will give your brain a boost for the day. Most new mothers don't have the time to sit down and have three meals a day, so try to graze or eat small meals throughout the day. Keep easy snacks in your refrigerator that are high in protein and that you can grab with one hand. This will help increase your energy and brain health.

Brain-Friendly Foods

Eat brain-friendly foods to improve brain performance. Not only will a diet full of brain-nourishing food (see below) have a positive effect on your brain function, but it will also give you the energy that you need to care for your newborn and yourself. The foods listed below will help you sleep better, give you strength and energy, and make you feel a whole lot better in general (Zuniga & McAuley, 2015).

Healthy fats, such as olive oil, nuts, and seeds (especially walnuts), flaxseed, and avocados are all good for promoting brain health (Ganzer & Zauderer, 2011). Cook with olive oil or use it on salad. You can combine it with balsamic vinegar or tamari sauce. Adding avocado (a fatty fruit) to your salad is a great way to add taste along with a mono-saturated fat to your salad or sandwich. Avocados can help your blood to flow, which adds to brain health (Johnson, Vishwanathan, Mohn, Haddock, Rasmussen, & Scott, 2015). They also help to lower blood pressure, which also contributes to a healthy brain.

Nuts and seeds are good sources of Vitamin E, which is an antioxidant that helps to keep membranes and cells healthy. Vitamin E has been shown to help preserve brain function and improve cognition (Zuniga & McAuley, 2015). Sources such as almonds, sunflower seeds, sesame seeds, hazelnuts, Brazil nuts, cashews, and walnuts are all good for your brain health. Purchasing natural, raw nuts is best. Unsalted roasted nuts are better for you than salted and roasted, and have fewer calories as well. Nuts are quick and easy to eat, and you can take them with you wherever you go.

You can purchase nut butters, such as almond butter, sunflower seed butter, cashew butter, and tahini, which is made from sesame seeds. Some of these nuts, such as almonds and sesame seeds, also contain calcium, which is good for your bones. Not only do these make healthy snacks, they are also good on the go. You can buy small packets of nuts or make your own trail mix and keep it handy in a small Ziplock bag. Other healthy snacks include raisins, fruit, yogurt, nutrition bars that are low in sugar and chemical ingredients (such as granola, Kindbar, Larabar, or Luna bars), cubes of cheese, carrot sticks, hard boiled eggs, string cheese, rice cakes, and small sandwiches on whole grain bread. These are all snacks you can keep in Ziplock bags in the refrigerator, so you can throw them in the diaper bag if you are running out. Some of them (for example, nuts, bars, or trail mix), you can even keep in your car.

Lean proteins, such as fish, lean meats, poultry, eggs, and soy are all packed with protein, are low in fat, and can give you lots of energy and stamina. Fish high in omega-3 fatty acids has also been shown to benefit brain health. Cold-water fish contains valuable levels of omega-3 fatty acids, and includes halibut, mackerel, salmon, trout, and tuna (Urwin, Miles, Noakes, Kremmyda, Vlachava, Diaper, & Yaqoob, 2012). Wild salmon is preferred over farmed salmon, because it tends to have higher levels of long-chain omega-3 fatty acids (EPA) than farm-raised salmon. Salmon is very high in omega-3s (EPA and DHA), which is very important for brain function. Sardines are also very high in the omega-3 (EPA) and are good for your brain as well (Farr, Price, Dominguez, Motisi, Saiano, Niehoff, & Barbagallo, 2012; Féart, Samieri, Rondeau et al, 2009; Seetharaman et al., 2015).

Antioxidants have been shown to decrease inflammation and help improve cognitive function in the brain. Fruits and vegetables are a source of naturally occurring antioxidants. High levels of this important compound can be found in vegetables such as kale, spinach, Brussel sprouts, alfalfa sprouts, broccoli, beets, red bell peppers, onions, and eggplant. Dark-skinned fruits with high antioxidant content include prunes, raisins, blueberries, blackberries, strawberries, raspberries, plums, oranges, red grapes, and cherries.

Blueberries, in particular, contain anthocyanosides, a compound proven to prevent harm caused by free radicals in the brain; they have also been shown to slow down oxidative stress, which is the imbalance between the body's production of free radicals, and the body's ability to detoxify their harmful effects (Krikorian, Shidler, Nash, Kalt, Vinqvist-Tymchuk, Shukitt-Hale, & Joseph, 2010). One cup a day is recommended. Blueberries can be eaten fresh, frozen, or freeze-dried. Throw a cup full of frozen blueberries into a smoothie with milk, or almond or soymilk, a tablespoon of nut butter, some protein powder (such as Spirutein, or Jay Robbs whey or egg protein), and you have a meal on the go!

"Wear" Your Newborn

There are many apparatuses on the market today for babies, such as baby swings, bouncy seats, rockers, activity gyms and play mats, jumpers, rock and play, pack and play, tummy time mats, piano gyms, rocking swings, and many others. All of these contraptions push your newborn away from you. Your newborn has been with you for nine months. He knows your every move, your heartbeat, your breathing, and your voice. Chances are when you put your newborn baby down, he will cry. Your baby wants to be with you, not away from you in an unfamiliar object, no matter how bright and colorful it is. Your newborn wants to feel your warmth and have familiar mom close by. Of course, you can't have your newborn under your bathrobe doing skin-to-skin contact all day long, but there are other ways to hold your newborn close to you while freeing you up a bit.

There are many devices that are intended for carrying your baby, also known as "baby wearing." The practice of wearing your baby has been around for centuries. Mothers used to wrap their infants in shawls, or any type of sling, so that they could get their household chores completed and care for older children. This practice allows you to hold your newborn close to you while getting things done around the house or while outdoors. Infants love feeling the rocking and movement of your everyday life.

There are many different types of infant slings and most are relatively inexpensive. You can also create your own, as long as you are sure it is safe, it doesn't obstruct breathing, and the baby can't fall out. Some slings are quite decorative and have a variety of styles, colors, and patterns. There are front carriers, back carriers, wrap carriers, and sling carriers. Brands include Baby Bjorn, Momwrap, Mobywrap, Ergobaby, the Peanut shell, Balboa baby, Karma baby—the list goes on. You can get these wraps in any baby store, as well as any baby superstore, or online. This is all you need for the first six weeks. Keep your newborn close to you and you both will be happy, comfortable, and secure.

The Juggling Act

Try to reduce tasks and spend time on what matters most: taking care of yourself and being with your newborn. Don't run around frenzied all day doing errands and other things. The first six weeks after giving birth are probably the most difficult weeks of your life. You can't expect to function the way you did before you had your baby. You need to give yourself a break from all of the juggling of activities that you normally do. Caring for yourself and your newborn should be your top priority—everything else can wait for right now. Accept meals from people, and offers of help from friends and family members. Do less. Ask more—sometimes people don't know what to do to help. Don't be too intimidated to ask for simple things. If a friend asks if she could stop by and visit, you can ask her to bring you something that you need—milk, eggs, or even a latte and a muffin. Don't feel as if you have to do it all.

This is the time to stay in your pajamas with your newborn in close contact, and nurture yourself, your mind, and your body. These six weeks can be a time for recuperation if you allow them to be. You are learning and healing, and you will never get this precious time back. Don't overload yourself or your brain, and don't expect to do everything you did before, or look exactly the same. If you appear to be out and about and functioning as before, no one will realize you need help and probably won't offer it.

Also, be good to your brain. Too much information and stress can cause it to become overloaded. Try not to multitask too much. Experience living in the moment, and enjoying every aspect of your first six weeks as a new mother. The more time you spend with your newborn, the faster and better the two of you will become in-sync. You will learn when he is tired, wet, hungry, or just plain fussy. Slow down your pace and in a few months (not in the first six weeks) you will be able to feel like yourself again.

Giving birth to your newborn is the biggest transformation of your life, and you will never be the same—in a good way!

Resources

Baby Center
www.babycenter.com

Café Mom
www.cafemom.com

Healthy Mom & Baby
www.health4mom.org

Holistic Mamas: Because Mother Nature knows best
www.holisticmamas.com

New Mother New Baby
www.newmothernewbaby.com

Chapter 2
Post-Baby Body

"This is not my body!"
"Whose body is this?"
"What has happened to my body?"

You were probably surprised at all the changes you experienced during your pregnancy. Your entire body has been affected in some way, from your hair, all the way down to your feet. But what exactly happens to your body after the birth of your baby?

The Four Stages of Labor

Labor has four stages. The first stage begins when your labor contractions start and ends when your cervix is completely thinned (effaced) and open (dilated). This stage consists of three parts (or phases): early, active, and transition. Once the cervix is fully dilated (10 centimeters), you enter the second stage of labor where your baby is ready to be pushed out into the world! If you delivered vaginally, you will remember this stage very well. You had to work hard, together with your contractions, to push your baby out. This second stage of labor begins when the cervix is completely thinned and open (fully dilated) and ends with the birth of the baby. This is also known as the *pushing stage*.

You may vaguely remember after the birth of your baby, someone telling you to push yet again! This last push was for the placenta. This is the third stage of labor and it begins with the birth of the baby and ends with the birth of the placenta. This is also known as the *placental stage*.

The fourth stage of labor, also known as the *recovery stage*, begins with the birth of the placenta, and typically ends once your body has stabilized (Durham & Chapman, 2014; Pillitteri, 2014; Ricci et al., 2013; Rice-Simpson & Creehan, 2014).

Many health care providers consider this period to extend for about six to eight weeks. This is the period of time from your baby's birth until your body makes an almost complete recovery. This is known as the postpartum period, or the *puerperium,* which means the period of time following childbirth.

What Happens to Your Body During Postpartum Period?

It is during this stage that your body, hormones, and uterus will readjust to not being pregnant. It takes about six weeks, sometimes longer, for your reproductive organs to return to their non-pregnant state (Durham & Chapman, 2014; Pillitteri, 2014; Ricci et al., 2013, Rice-Simpson & Creehan, 2014).

Notice how I say non-pregnant and not pre-pregnant. The reason for this is that once you deliver a baby, your organs, your muscles, and bone structure (e.g., hips) will have changed slightly, and do not return to your pre-pregnancy state. This is not a bad thing; your body, after all, has created your beautiful baby! Your body will change in a number of ways. Your body on the inside, and possibly on the outside as well, will be a little bit different after birth. Labor and birth affects almost all of the body systems, which is why it is important for you to rest and listen to your body during this time. If you give your body a chance to heal itself, you are helping to avoid any unforeseen complications.

Postpartum Recovery

What types of changes happen?
When will things go back to normal?
How long will it take for me to recover?
Is there anything I can do to make
the recovery quicker and easier?

All new mothers recover at different rates and experience different types of symptoms depending on how their pregnancy and birth took place.

Many different factors can affect the way you will heal during this time. It is important to give yourself time to recuperate, get to know your baby, and be aware of any signs of complications. Oftentimes a new mother will push herself to get her life and body back as soon as possible after the baby's birth, experiencing spurts of energy and the desire to "do it all!" You may have a lot of emotional energy, and it can be very tempting to want to get the house back in order, grocery shop, cook, or run around returning or exchanging baby gifts. You may want to prepare yourself for returning to work by taking care of errands and household chores that you will not get to do once you return to your job.

The reality is that your body has gone through a tremendous ordeal. You have had major changes happen to your body, emotions, and hormones. That's not even counting the actual birth! Whether you had a vaginal birth, or a cesarean birth, your body has still been stretched and torn, and you produced a baby. Please don't take this lightly— this was not a small thing that you did. Birth is a life changing event. It took nine months for you to grow your baby, and many hours of labor and birth. Now is the time to let your body heal.

Your mind and emotions will follow along with your healing. Your body will heal faster if you take care of yourself by resting as much as you can, eating healthy foods throughout the day, and drinking plenty of fluids, especially water. As previously mentioned, having some help for the first few days or weeks will do wonders for your recovery. If you start running around and doing too much, you may feel more fatigued in the long run, which can make your recovery take that much longer. You can also develop complications, such as increased bleeding, anemia, infection, or gastrointestinal problems.

This is your time to bond with your newborn, relax, watch television, read, and let someone else do the shopping and cooking, or order food in. You will never have this time back again, so take full advantage of it. Your body will soon let you know if you are doing too much.

Don't be in a hurry to get back into shape. Try not to compare yourself with celebrities who have their bodies back a month after they had their baby. They have unusual circumstances, money for hired help, trainers, and someone to prepare food for them. They may have also undergone surgery to remove excess skin or fat from their abdomens. These women take extraordinary means to get their bodies back into shape, as their careers and livelihood depend on their appearance. For the average new mom, it takes more time. More important than losing the baby weight is that you eat a healthy, balanced diet, and exercise moderately when your body is ready. You need to be rested and healthy in order to have the energy to care for yourself and your newborn.

Post-Baby Pelvic Organs

How long will it take for my uterus to shrink back to normal?

The physical changes you will be experiencing after the birth of your baby can be quite surprising. Having a better understanding of what is happening to your body will help you cope better, and help you to take the steps you need towards proper healing.

The pre-pregnant uterus is a lot smaller than you think! It rests deep within your abdomen, in between your bladder and rectum. Before pregnancy, it is shaped like an upside-down pear. The top part of the uterus is called the *fundus,* and the bottom part of the uterus is called

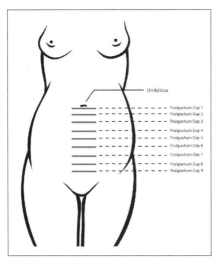

the *cervix.* As your pregnancy progressed, your uterus had grown upward and outward. By the end of nine months, your uterus will have looked like an inflated balloon. Immediately after your baby was born and the placenta was expelled, your uterus began to shrink. This shrinking, or contracting, is called the involution process (Durham & Chapman, 2014; Pillitteri, 2014; Ricci et al., 2013; Rice-Simpson & Creehan, 2014).

The area inside your uterus from where the placenta was attached also needs to heal. The first few days after your baby's birth you can actually feel the top part of your uterus, the *fundus,* a little bit below your belly button (navel). It will feel firm and round, and be about the size of a grapefruit. During your hospital or birthing-center stay, the nurses and other health care providers were feeling for your fundus and massaging it to make sure that it was contracting and remaining firm. If the fundus is soft, or what we call "boggy," there is a chance for heavy bleeding, which may lead to a hemorrhage. By remaining firm, your vaginal bleeding will be under control and your fundus will slowly reduce in size each day. It will descend back down into the pelvis by about one-half inch per day (Durham & Chapman, 2014; Pillitteri, 2014; Ricci et al., 2013; Rice- Simpson, & Creehan, 2014).

Each day, your uterus will decrease in height. By ten days, you will no longer be able to feel your fundus from the outside of your abdomen. This process will happen faster in the breastfeeding woman, and slower after a caesarean birth. If you gave birth to twins, triplets, or more or if you already birthed more than three or four children in the past, you will experience a slower involution process. If your uterus is not shrinking, there may be an infection or possibly some blood or tissue from the delivery that was not flushed out during the birth. If you continue to have bright red bleeding after your third postpartum day, notify your health care provider (Durham, & Chapman, 2014; Pillitteri, 2014; Ricci et al., 2013; Rice-Simpson & Creehan, 2014).

What are these cramp-like pains I am having?
Why are they worse when I breastfeed?

These are known as "after pains," and they may become quite uncomfortable. You may feel some cramping as the process of involution is taking place. This is a good sign and indicates that your uterus is contracting properly and getting back to the location it is supposed to be in your non-pregnant body. Your uterus is working hard to contract and return to its non-pregnant state. These pains will feel like strong menstrual cramps, and sometimes they can be as strong as a labor contraction. The strength of these contractions varies between new mothers. First-time mothers usually do not experience very strong afterbirth pains. A mother who has had her second or third baby will usually experience more discomfort. The reason for this is that the uterus has been stretched already. It has to work harder to get back to its normal shape and size after the second or third baby than it does after the first baby.

You may not feel the urge to urinate due to the physical trauma of your birth, but it is important for you to try and empty your bladder frequently. If your bladder is full, it can cause your uterus to be displaced to the side, preventing it from contracting. If you experience a sudden gush of heavy bleeding and strong cramping, try emptying your bladder first. This will allow your uterus to go back to its center position, and then the bleeding should be under control. Seeing that sudden gush of blood can be frightening. If it continues after your bladder is empty, please notify your health care provider.

If your afterbirth pains become very uncomfortable, they can be relieved by using a hot water bottle, heating pad, or an over-the-counter pain reliever, such as acetaminophen (Tylenol) or ibuprofen (Motrin, Advil). If you are breastfeeding, the pain reliever should be taken approximately one hour before the baby feeds to allow your body to metabolize the medication and provide more comfort for you while you are breastfeeding. Staying on top of the pain by taking your medication at regular intervals, as prescribed, rather than as needed, is a good idea in the beginning. Once the pain sets in, it can build rather quickly, and it can be more difficult to get the pain under control. This technique will actually decrease your use of pain medication in the long run, rather than increase its use. You can also contact your health care provider for a prescription pain reliever if you feel that you need something stronger (Durham & Chapman, 2014; Pillitteri, 2014; Ricci et al., 2013; Rice-Simpson & Creehan, 2014).

Post-Baby Bleeding (Lochia)

Is it normal to bleed after delivery?
What exactly is Lochia?
How much is normal?

The vaginal bleeding you will experience after your baby's birth can be quite different than the normal menstrual cycle that you are used to. This bleeding is a discharge called *lochia*. It is a combination of blood, mucus, and post-birth tissue that is being cleared from your uterus as the lining of your uterus goes through the healing process. In the first few days after birth, your bleeding can be quite heavy, and you may experience some clots as well. When you stand up after you have been lying in bed or sitting in a chair, you may experience a gush of blood. This can be very frightening, but it is perfectly normal and is caused by an accumulation, or pooling, of the blood while you were lying down. As long as you are not regularly bleeding or soaking through more than one pad per hour, with large clots, there is no need to be concerned (Durham & Chapman, 2014; Pillitteri, 2014; Ricci et al., 2013; Rice-Simpson, & Creehan, 2014).

How can I tell if I am bleeding too much?

Medically speaking, your bleeding will be classified as follows:

- **Scant:** if there is less than 1 inch of a spot of blood across the pad
- **Light:** if there is less than 4 inches of a spot of blood across the pad
- **Moderate:** if there is less than 6 inches of a spot of blood across the pad
- **Heavy:** if the entire pad is saturated with blood after one hour

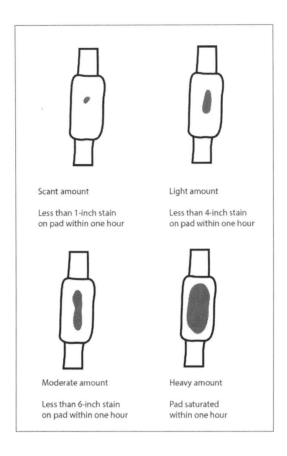

Scant amount

Less than 1-inch stain
on pad within one hour

Light amount

Less than 4-inch stain
on pad within one hour

Moderate amount

Less than 6-inch stain
on pad within one hour

Heavy amount

Pad saturated
within one hour

For the new mother, these are estimates, and any bleeding that you sense is abnormal should be brought to the attention of your health care provider. The best pads during this time would be maxi overnight pads. Make sure you purchase the unscented pads, as you do not want chemicals to be around your vaginal area while your cervix is still open. You also may have stitches in your perineal area, and you do not want to irritate them or cause an infection. Remember that tampons are not to be used under any circumstances. If you find that you are soaking through one pad per hour, and the color is bright red and contains large clots, notify your health care provider.

How long will the bleeding last?

If everything proceeds normally and without complications, your lochia will change in color, amount, and consistency over the next 6 weeks. You can expect the following: a dark red-colored lochia, known as *lochia rubra*, for the first 2 to 3 days; a brownish discharge called *lochia serosa* for the next 7 days (days 3 to 10); and finally, a yellowish discharge called *lochia alba* for the next 3 to 6 weeks. This pattern can vary from new mother to new mother, and with each baby you birth.

I mentioned earlier that your body needs rest so it can heal. Not resting can have a direct impact on your bleeding cycle. Sometimes the dark-red bleeding can stop for a few days or weeks, and then suddenly return. This is your body's way of letting you know that you are doing too much. If you take a step back and take it easy, the bleeding will stop and return to the *lochia serosa* or *alba* that you may have had originally at that time. Normal lochia will have an odor of fresh blood. It is very important if you notice a foul smell from your lochia, a heavier than usual flow, continuous large clots, chills, or fever, to notify your health care provider. These symptoms can be a sign of infection or other complication (Durham & Chapman, 2014; Pillitteri, 2014; Ricci et al., 2013; Rice-Simpson & Creehan, 2014).

Warning Signs

- Your lochia is bright red, or has returned to bright red after becoming pink, 4 days after birth.

- Your lochia has a strong, foul odor and/or you develop fever or chills.

- You have very heavy bleeding (saturating one pad per hour pad and/or large blood clots bigger than a quarter).

- Copious amounts of bleeding, and/or feeling dizzy, or faint.

With any of these signs, please call your health care provider or go to the nearest emergency department, as you may be having a postpartum hemorrhage.

Post-Baby Cervix

What exactly is a cervix?
What is its role during birth and postpartum?

Your cervix is considered to be the opening to the womb. Your cervix is a very small organ at the bottom part of your uterus. It connects the vagina to the uterus and it is shaped like a tube. It is often called the "neck" of the uterus, and it opens into the vagina. It is about 1 ½ to 2 inches long, 1 inch wide, and plays a crucial role during labor and birth. There is a small opening inside the cervix called the *os*, which allows your menstrual blood to flow through when you are not pregnant. During your pregnancy, your cervix will be completely closed, holding inside of it a plug of mucus that is protecting the baby from outside bacteria. As the cervix thins and opens up, the mucus plug is expelled, breaking off some of the small capillaries. The combination of the blood from the broken capillaries and the mucus from the plug is the pink discharge you had seen before your labor began, and is known as "bloody show" (Durham, & Chapman, 2014; Pillitteri, 2014; Ricci et al., 2013; Rice-Simpson, & Creehan, 2014).

Your cervix, once it had opened and thinned out completely, allowed your baby to pass through your uterus, into your vagina, and out of your body. Your cervix may be swollen and bruised. It has also been stretched and distended. It will begin to close immediately after birth, and will return to a normal size and position by about 6 weeks. It will also be healing from the trauma of the birth during this time. After a vaginal delivery, the center of the cervix (*os*) will change in shape slightly. Instead of a small hole in the middle of the cervix, there will be a slit. This is called a "fish mouth." If you have not had a vaginal delivery, your cervix will remain the same as before: a small circular hole.

Post-Baby Vagina

How much will my vagina be stretched after I give birth?
Did childbirth damage my vagina?

Your vagina will have gone through some minor trauma, and in some circumstances, major trauma. If you are having continuous bleeding, or a slow trickle of blood, you must notify your health care provider, as there may be a tear in the vaginal tissue. After you give birth to a baby vaginally, your vagina will be slightly larger than it was before. How much larger depends on the size of your baby, and the number of babies you have had. Your pelvic floor muscles have been stretched to allow the baby to pass through the birth canal, and the muscles may have lost some tone. All of the pelvic organs will gradually begin to shrink back to their original sizes. However, it is normal for the vagina to be slightly larger than it was prior to giving birth.

Kegel exercises, also known as pelvic-floor exercises, are an excellent way to tighten the vaginal muscles (Lim, Barnett-Lopez, & Francisco, 2004). These exercises can also be beneficial if you are experiencing any leakage of urine, which most of the time, is only temporary. Kegel exercises will also help to tone the pelvic-floor muscles, and increase blood flow to the perineum, helping the healing process if you had an episiotomy or tear. By toning the vaginal and pelvic-floor muscles, your vagina will feel firmer, and as a result, you may be able to enjoy sex more. Kegel exercises can be done anytime, anywhere, and no one knows you are doing them.

The first thing you need to do is to identify the muscles that you will be working on, which are your pelvic floor muscles. One way to identify pelvic-floor muscles is while urinating. Make an attempt to try and stop the flow of urine midstream. If you can hold the urine back, you have located the correct muscles. Then you can strengthen these muscles at any time of the day by tightening the pelvic floor and holding for a count of five, gradually increasing until ten. You can visualize the following scenario: an elevator climbing up three to four floors, making the muscles tighter and tighter at each floor. Once you reach the top floor, hold for a count of ten and then gradually release the tension, and go back down the floors, all the way to the basement, where the pelvic floor is completely relaxed. Do this as many times a day as you can remember. Try to set a specific time that you will remember to do these exercises, for example: when you are in the car, watching television, or feeding the baby.

There is a device on the market called a Kegelmaster that can help you identify these muscles and add resistance while strengthening and toning them. This device can only be used after the first six weeks, or when your health care provider gives you the okay. It is relatively inexpensive, easy to use, and can be ordered online. Biofeedback can also be used to gain more conscious control of your pelvic floor muscles. Biofeedback can actually measure the amount of muscle activity you are exerting and help you perform your Kegel exercises more effectively.

Post-Baby Perineal Pain

What is a perineum?
Why am I so sore?
When will my sutures heal?

Your perineum is the region of your body that is located between your vagina and your rectum. This is the area that may or may not have to be cut in order to allow more room for your baby to pass through. This procedure is called an *episiotomy*. It is a surgical incision that is made under a local anesthetic that your health care provider will inject into your skin as the baby is crowning (the baby's head is visible at the opening of the vagina).

If you did not have an episiotomy, your perineal area has still been stretched out and somewhat traumatized and therefore you may still have some soreness. If you had an episiotomy, you will be experiencing a bit more discomfort. You would have been given ice packs right after delivery for the first 24 hours. Usually, a new mother is given topical pain medications after delivery, and you can continue using them when you get home (Durham & Chapman, 2014; Pillitteri, 2014; Ricci et al., 2013; Rice- Simpson & Creehan, 2014).

There are many over-the-counter helpful remedies that you can also try as long as your health care provider approves of them. Witch hazel pads are very soothing. I recommend lining up the witch hazel pads on the sanitary pad, and then keeping the pads in place until your next trip to the bathroom. You can also use a topical anesthetic spray, such as Dermoplast, on the area, along with the topical ointments you were given by your health care provider. Taking care to keep the incision clean is very important to prevent infection and allow for healing. Following these guidelines will help the healing process:

- ▸ Change your sanitary pad each time you urinate or use the bathroom, or at least every 4 hours.

- ▸ Continue to use the perineal bottle you were given at the hospital or birthing center to wash the area after you urinate. Pat the area dry (baby wipes are good for this), and be sure not to rub.

- ▸ Warm-water sitz baths (a warm-water bath covering the hips) can be very soothing. If you don't have a plastic sitz bath, you can fill the bathtub with a little warm water up to your hips or buttocks, and sit in it for at least 20 minutes at a time. Sitz baths are also good for hemorrhoids and are not only soothing to the affected area, but help to increase blood flow, allowing for faster healing.

- ▸ If it hurts to sit, you can sit on a pillow, a donut (a pillow with a hole cut out), or an inflated tube.

- ▸ Wear loose clothing over the area.

- ▸ Try Kegel exercises (see above). These exercises allow for circulation of blood flow to the area to promote healing and increase muscle tone.

You may need a pain reliever, or an anti-inflammatory medication, for your discomfort. Some women will need something even stronger than that. Talk to your health care provider if you feel that the over-the-counter medications are not working for you. She can prescribe other medications, such as Percocet (oxycodone and acetaminophen) or Tylenol (acetaminophen) with Codeine, which can help relieve your discomfort (Durham & Chapman, 2014).

Be patient. Healing times vary and can take up to 6 weeks and, in some situations, longer. The deeper the tear or episiotomy, the longer it will take to heal. You may feel some soreness for up to 4 to 6 months. Please call your health care provider if you are feeling continuous perineal pain after the first few days, increased swelling in the area, or if you have a fever of more than 100 degrees Fahrenheit.

Post-Baby Bladder

Why am I sweating so much?
Why is it so hard for me to urinate?

After birth, your body will eliminate a lot of fluids that you had been retaining during pregnancy. Your body no longer needs these fluids and you will be flushing out large amounts of urine as a result. You will also be sweating a lot during the first few postpartum days. This is known as postpartum diuresis and is a result of the drop in pregnancy hormones. These sweating episodes tend to occur during the night. You may wake up drenched in sweat. If this happens, it is a good idea to change your pajamas so you do not become chilled.

If you have had an epidural or another type of anesthesia, your bladder may be temporarily swollen and have less muscle tone. You may experience a reduced sensation in the bladder area as a result. You may not feel your bladder as being full in this case, or you may have some difficulty urinating at first. These sensations will usually decrease after 24 hours. Your bladder may have also been a bit traumatized by the birth and you may not feel the urge as you used to. Having had an epidural during labor may have decreased your sensation in the area (Durham & Chapman, 2014; Pillitteri, 2014; Ricci et al., 2013; Rice-Simpson & Creehan, 2014).

How can I help to ease the discomfort
in the perineal area and help the urine flow better?

Use the following suggestions:

- ▸ Use your peri bottle to spray warm water on your perineal area. This will help to stimulate the flow of urine and ease the discomfort if you had an episiotomy.

- ▸ Try listening to the flow of running water if you are having difficulty urinating.

- ▸ A warm sitz bath can also help with the flow of urine, either the plastic one you may have received from the hospital or birthing center, or you can make your own by sitting in a tub filled with a little bit of warm water (no soap).

- ▸ Drink lots of fluids, especially water, to dilute the urine and help flush out toxins. This can also help with constipation, which can disrupt the flow of urine.

Any pain or burning sensation when urinating can be a sign of a urinary tract infection (UTI). If this occurs, notify your health care provider. It is very important to try and empty your bladder completely to prevent a UTI. If your urine output is less than normal for yourself, or you have difficulty urinating, call your health care provider. Typically, the renal system will return to normal by 6 weeks postpartum.

Why am I leaking urine sometimes?
Why do I have the urge to urinate so often?

Urinary incontinence can be quite common after giving birth not only due to the trauma your pelvic-floor muscles have experienced, but also due to the weakening of the muscles surrounding the bladder and pelvis. This is most likely temporary, but can take anywhere from 3 to 6 months to resolve (Lim, Barnett-Lopez, & Fancisco, 2004).

The following techniques can help you regain bladder control:

- ▸ Kegel exercises can help regain muscle tone, thereby helping to control the bladder muscles.

- ▶ Avoid bladder irritants, such as coffee (even decaf), citrusy or acidic fruits and juices (such as oranges, grapefruits, and tomatoes), sodas, and alcohol.

- ▶ Drink lots of clear fluids, water, or herbal teas to help flush out toxins and keep things moving smoothly.

- ▶ Avoid constipation, which can cause you to strain and add extra weight and stress to your bladder.

- ▶ Try bladder training. Empty your bladder every half hour or so and gradually increase the time that you urinate. Try not to urinate out of habit. Only when you need to.

- ▶ Wear a pad in case of leaking until things are under control.

- ▶ There are medications that your health care provider can prescribe temporarily to decrease spasms of the bladder and retrain your bladder to contract better and hold more urine.

- ▶ Biofeedback exercises can help control bladder muscles. You will need to go to a specialist who provides biofeedback specifically for bladder control.

Post-Baby Belly

Why do I still look five months pregnant?
Will I ever have a flat stomach again?

You may be quite surprised that you still look pregnant during your first 6 weeks postpartum. There are several reasons for this. Remember the inflated balloon we compared your uterus to at the end of your pregnancy? Now that your baby is out of your uterus, the balloon will need to deflate. This happens more as a slow leak rather than an eruption as if a pin pricked it. As a result, your uterus is still enlarged and does not return to a non-pregnant state for 6 weeks. It took 9 months for your body to stretch, and it will take time for it to reduce in size. The ligaments surrounding your uterus have been stretched and need the entire 6 weeks for full recovery.

Even though your baby is out of your uterus, your uterus is still enlarged and will take 6 weeks for it to contract back to its original size. You are also retaining fluids, which your body will flush out over the next few weeks through urine and sweating. Your abdomen will be distended, with some sagging skin—this is completely normal. You abdominal muscles and the skin surrounding the abdomen have been stretched to accommodate the size of your baby along with all the other components of your pregnancy. Your muscle tone is decreased and your muscles have become soft and relaxed. Over time, with exercise, your muscles will regain their tone.

Some of you may develop a separation of the abdominal muscle during pregnancy. This is known as a *diastasis*. A diastasis is a separation of the outer abdominal muscles, which support your organs and your back. Your muscles, therefore, are weakened. This condition can be improved with exercise.

Stretch marks, also called *striae,* are a result of the stretching and breakage of your skin's elastic threads. The color of your striae may be red or purple, but eventually will fade to a silvery whitish color. There are many products on the market that may help to reduce your scarring, such as cocoa butter. It is important to remember not to get too caught up with weight loss, especially in the first 6 weeks. It is not worth injuring yourself, or making yourself sick, in order to get back into shape quickly. It takes time for the rest of the baby weight to come off, and it takes time for your body to heal and get back into shape. Your body needs to heal so you can be strong enough to care for your baby.

Post-Baby Breasts

Will my breasts ever be the same after birth?

Your breasts have been preparing for birth and lactation by undergoing many changes throughout the pregnancy. Fullness and swelling of the breasts are normal during pregnancy and the first couple of days after birth. Between the second and fifth day, all postpartum women, whether they are breastfeeding or not, will experience a more extreme fullness. Your breasts will become larger, firmer, heavier, warm, and more sensitive (International Lactation Consultant Association, 2013, for more details, see Chapter 4, Post-Baby Breastfeeding and Breast Care).

Post-Baby Digestion

Why do I have so much gas, bloating, back and abdominal pain?
How am I supposed to have a bowel movement with stitches
and pain "down there?"

Your gastrointestinal system will return to normal shortly after birth. This is mostly because your enlarged uterus is no longer putting pressure on all of the organs in your abdomen. However, this does take time, and most women will have a lazy bowel for the first few days. Medications, surgery, not enough fluids, and reduced muscle tone can be the reason for this. You may be afraid to have a bowel movement if you had an episiotomy, tears, or hemorrhoids, or you may try to postpone it or ignore the urge. Hemorrhoids may have been present during the pregnancy, or may have been pushed out of the rectum during the pushing stage of labor. Constipation is very common during this time (for more information, see Chapter 6, Post-Baby Diet and Nutrition).

Post-Baby Joints

Is it normal to have joint and muscle aches after birth?
Will it go away?

Your muscles and joints have all been affected during your pregnancy. The hormones of pregnancy, estrogen, progesterone, and relaxin all have an effect on your joints, causing them to become more relaxed. Weight gain during pregnancy can also throw off the center of gravity for a lot of women making them more clumsy and vulnerable to falls or accidents. After birth, these hormones decrease and the joints and muscles return back to normal by 6 weeks postpartum. Some women may notice at this point that their shoe size has increased. Initially, this may be due to swelling. But many women experience a permanent increase in shoe size after birth. As these hormones are slowing down, you may feel tired, and may have some hip and joint pain. This is why it is a good idea to wait 6 weeks before beginning any rigorous exercise program, when the muscles and joints have calmed down and have become more stable.

Post-Baby Skin and Hair

Why is my hair falling out?
Is this normal?
Will it grow back?
When will it stop?

Again, the hormones estrogen and progesterone play a role in skin and hair changes throughout your pregnancy and postpartum period. You may have noticed a darkened line down the abdomen known as *linea nigra*. You may have also noticed an increased number of freckles or a darkened area across your nose and cheeks, known as *chloasma*. These pigments will fade gradually over the next few months.

During pregnancy, hormones caused your hair and nails to become stronger. Estrogen triggered a prolonged growth phase causing your hair to appear thicker and fuller. You were probably very happy and excited about this. However, after birth, when your hormones are decreasing, the hair you did not lose during pregnancy will begin to shed. You may be losing more hair than usual. This may not happen for a few months, but you may notice excess hair in your hairbrush, shower, or you may find it in your hands after touching your hair. This can be very disturbing, as your hair may appear thinner than it was before the pregnancy. Try not to be too concerned; you will not lose all of your hair. Within a few months, your hair will be back to normal. For some new mothers, the hair texture will also change slightly. Here are some tips you can try to diminish your hair loss and make yourself feel and look better:

▶ Continue taking prenatal vitamins; eat a well-balanced diet with plenty of protein, fruits, and vegetables. This will help you nourish your hair, as hair is a protein and can make the hair loss decrease and help your hair look fuller and thicker.

► Try a thickening shampoo; there are many shampoos that add volume to the hair. Some products also have protein in them, which can help your hair feel fuller and thicker. Try not to use a heavy conditioner, as this can weigh down the hair. Use conditioners specific for fine hair, or only apply the conditioner to the ends.

► Postpone any type of coloring or any chemical treatments. Avoid blow-drying, curling, straightening, too much brushing, scrunchies, or clips as these can pull on the hair and cause more hair loss.

► Try a new shorter hairstyle that can make your hair appear thicker and fuller.

Post-Baby Menstruation

When will I get my period again?
Can I get pregnant during this time?
Will breastfeeding prevent pregnancy?

It must have been a nice break for you to not have your period for nine months. It will soon be back, and may be heavier and last longer than before your pregnancy. After the birth of your baby and the placenta, pregnancy hormones, estrogen and progesterone, immediately stop production. For the new mother who is either bottle-feeding or not breastfeeding exclusively, you may resume normal hormonal changes that go along with ovulation. The lochia you will be experiencing for 4 to 6 weeks is not your menstrual cycle; it is the byproducts of conception. For the bottle-feeding mother, your menstrual cycle may begin again in about 2 to 3 months. For the breastfeeding mother, this usually takes a bit longer. Your cycle may resume in 3 to 4 months, or it may not return for up to a year (Durham & Chapman, 2014; Pillitteri, 2014; Ricci et al., 2013; Rice- Simpson & Creehan, 2014).

A breastfeeding mother who exclusively breastfeeds around the clock can delay ovulation. Breastfeeding's effect on fertility, and as a method of family planning, has been studied extensively. This approach prompted a method of family planning called the lactation amenorrhea method (LAM). The principle of LAM is that a woman who continues to exclusively breastfeed her newborn, around the clock, and does not begin to menstruate during her first 6 months postpartum, is protected from pregnancy during that time. These studies have supported LAM as an acceptable method of birth control. When using this method, you need to be cautious; if you begin to menstruate prior to 6 months postpartum, continue to breastfeed after 6 months, use any supplemental feedings, or do not feed your newborn during the night, you run the risk of becoming pregnant, and therefore should use a backup method of birth control (Gray, Campbell, Apelo, Eslami, Zacur, Ramos, & Labbok, 1990; Perez, Labbok, & Queenan, 1992; For more details, see Chapter 7, Post-Baby Love and Sex).

Your cycle now may be quite different than prior to your pregnancy. Some women experience much heavier flows than they used to have before the pregnancy. Some women may experience premenstrual syndrome (PMS), even if they did not have it before pregnancy, and those that did, may experience a worsening of symptoms. Symptoms may include breast tenderness, fatigue, insomnia, mood swings, lower back pain, acne breakouts, bloating, weight gain, cravings, increased appetite, irritability, depression, anxiety, or crying spells. There are a variety of remedies that you can try for PMS if you find these symptoms unmanageable. Here are some lifestyle changes that can help.

- ► When your body has healed, and you get the okay from your health care provider, try to get as much exercise as you can. This can be difficult with a new baby. However, even taking the baby for a walk in the stroller for 20 minutes for a few days a week is good exercise.

- ► Eat a healthy diet, including fruits, vegetables, whole grains, and protein, and try to limit dairy products.

- ► Minimize sugar and caffeine. Both of these can make you anxious.

- ► Avoid tobacco and alcohol.

- ► Minimize salt intake one week prior to your cycle. Salt can increases swelling and bloating.

- ► Listening to relaxation tapes, or doing yoga or Pilates, can all help to decrease symptoms and promote wellness during this time.

- ► You can try using a heating pad or hot water bottle for abdominal discomfort.

- ► Journaling about your emotions and feelings can help put your thoughts into perspective for you, and give you an emotional outlet.

- ► Supplements, such as Vitamin B6 (50-100mg) can help reduce your symptoms of swelling and bloating. Vitamin B6 can mimic a natural diuretic.

- ► Vitamin D (1,000-3,000 IU), not only in the winter months, can help to improve your mood. It's a good idea to get your Vitamin D levels checked, as you may be deficient and need a higher dose than the one recommended.

- ► Vitamin E (400 IU) can help to reduce breast tenderness. Vitamin E is a fat-soluble vitamin that is an antioxidant and also reduces inflammation. It can help to reduce mild breast tenderness and swelling before cycles.

- ► Calcium, at least 1,000-1,200 mg per day, is the recommended dose, and is good for your bones in general. Taking calcium with magnesium can prevent constipation and also have a calming effect on you.

- ► Herbal supplements, such as black cohosh and chaste berry (except if breastfeeding), and Omega-3 fish oil can also be helpful in balancing your hormones, and help you with your physical and emotional symptoms. You need to check with an herbalist or natu-ropath for the correct dosing with these herbs.

▸ You can also try ibuprofen (Motrin, Advil) to relieve cramps and discomfort (http://www.womenshealth.gov, 2010).

You may have heard of pre-menstrual dysphoric disorder, abbreviated as PMDD. PMDD is a more severe form of PMS, and is not normal PMS. A woman who develops PMDD may experience some of the following symptoms:

▸ Severe mood swings, with increased irritability, anger, markedly depressed mood, hopelessness, marked anxiety, feeling as if on edge, feeling out of control, and lethargy.

▸ Difficulty concentrating, insomnia, or sleeping too much. A decrease in productivity at work, school, or home.

▸ Physical symptoms of bloating, muscle aches, joint pain, headaches and breast tenderness.

Symptoms occur about day 14 of your cycle (approximately one week prior to your period), and usually ease with the onset of your menstrual cycle (American Psychiatric Association, 2013). A decrease in the neurotransmitter, serotonin, may be a cause of PMDD. You can try any or all of the above remedies for PMS, or you may be prescribed an antidepressant, such as Prozac or Sarafem (fluoxetine), Zoloft (sertraline), Paxil (paroxetine), Celexa (citalopram), Lexapro (escitalopram), or Luvox (fluvoxamine). Some health care providers may prescribe a birth control pill if you are not breastfeeding, or the mini pill (Progesterone only) if you are breastfeeding. Taking oral contraceptives may help to regulate your mood swings, and can create a lighter menstrual flow. Be aware that some women may have an opposite reaction and have increased mood swings when taking oral contraceptives.

The changes that are taking place in your body, and in your home during the first 6 weeks can be very disrupting and overwhelming at first. Remember that this is your time to convalesce. If you let your body heal and take care of yourself, you will be better able to care for your baby. You have to learn your baby, and your baby has to learn you. Shutting out the rest of the world for now, and, caring for yourself and your baby, is the best thing you can do for the both of you during these 6 crucial weeks.

Resources

**Ask Dr. Sears:
The trusted resource
for parents**
www.askdrsears.com

**Café Mom:
The meeting place
for Moms**
www.cafemom.com

**KellyMom:
Evidence-based breast-
feeding and parenting**
www.kellymom.com

**Mothering: The home for
natural family living**
www.mothering.com

**Womenshealth.gov:
Office on women's health,
U.S. department of Health
and Human Services**
www.womenshealth.gov

**Women, Infants and
Children (WIC)**
www.health.ny.gov/prevention/
nutrition/wic/

Chapter 3
Post-Baby Cesarean Birth

"How long will it take for me to recover from my cesarean birth?"

"How is my recovery different than if I had a vaginal birth?"

A *cesarean birth* is the birth of a baby through an incision that is made in the abdomen and the uterus. It is also known as *cesarean section* or *cesarean delivery*, and is one of the oldest surgical procedures. A cesarean birth is also one of the most common major surgical procedures performed in the United States today. Cesarean section does carry more risk than a vaginal birth. Cesarean birth can be planned, performed after a Trial of Labor (TOL), which is a vaginal delivery attempt after a previous cesarean birth, or performed as an emergency. There are many medical reasons involving the mother, fetus, or the placenta that would necessitate a cesarean birth as opposed to a vaginal birth.

If you have had a cesarean birth, you will have more to handle when you go home with your newborn. You did not just give birth. You have given birth, and you have undergone major abdominal surgery. Having a newborn baby to take care of while recuperating from a surgical birth, along with the physical and emotional strain of it all, can be overwhelming. Even the simplest household tasks may seem monumental, such as getting into a comfortable position or lifting your newborn. Don't be afraid to ask for help. Keeping yourself as comfortable as possible will help you reduce your stress and you will be able to feed your newborn smoothly, whether by breast or bottle.

You will need to take time to rest and recuperate, and give your body a chance to heal. Enlist as much help as you possibly can. Allow yourself to be pampered and let others take care of you, so that you can take good care of your newborn. Let your body heal, rest, recover, and it will set you off to a good start. Taking good care of yourself in the first few weeks will help you to gain the strength and the confidence you need to be the best mother that you can be.

Cesarean Birth Recovery

You may have had a planned cesarean, which is considered elective, because you and your health care provider chose the date and planned it based on circumstances that would not have been advisable for you to have a vaginal delivery. Your cesarean birth would have been arranged according to your due date and the maturity of the fetus. You knew ahead of time that you would be having a cesarean birth. If this was the case, you would have had some time to plan—you may have even taken a childbirth class that specifically prepared you for a cesarean birth. If your cesarean birth had been planned, you would have had ample time to prepare yourself at home prior to going to the hospital. However, you will still feel somewhat sore and exhausted, and settling into a routine with your newborn may take more time than with a vaginal birth due to the effects of the surgery.

If your cesarean birth was an emergency, you probably did not have sufficient time to prepare for the birth. You may have been in labor for a very long time, or were pushing for several hours, and then had to have the baby delivered surgically. You may not be prepared for the recovery at home. An emergency cesarean birth is performed for reasons that arise suddenly in labor. These reasons can include problems with the placenta, fetus, or the labor not progressing. An emergency cesarean birth will have the same risks as a planned one. There are no additional risks other than the fact that the new mother—you—was not psychologically prepared. You may also be physically and emotionally exhausted from a lack of sleep and hours of labor. You may need to modify your original plans regarding help at home, maternity leave etc., when you return home with your newborn.

Regardless of the reason, you have now had a cesarean birth. You have undergone major surgery and your healing will be a little bit more involved than if you had a vaginal birth. Give your body the rest and care that it needs to heal. Not only have you had major surgery, but you also have a new baby to take care of. You will be processing all the emotional and physical factors of having surgery as well as making new adjustments in order to take good care of your newborn. You may be disappointed at having had a cesarean birth, and not be prepared for the after care. Or you may be happy that you had a planned birth, that you were able to prepare for it, and that you didn't have to experience labor. Or you may just be happy that your baby was born healthy, no matter which way he or she came out! If you are having a difficult time accepting your mode of delivery, there are many support groups that you can reach out to. There are also many support groups for Vaginal Birth After Cesarean (VBAC) if you wish to try to deliver your next baby vaginally, circumstances permitting.

After a cesarean birth, your hospital stay is about 3 or 4 days, maybe longer. By the time you come home from the hospital, your incision should be healing well on both the inside and outside. You may not be experiencing too much pain as the pain medication that you received in the hospital should have been working, and you may still be taking pain medication at home. You must be very careful not to do anything too strenuous, as the incision can open up. This would be a problem because any time an incision is infected or opens up; it forms scar tissue and takes longer to heal.

Indications for Cesarean Birth

Maternal

- ▸ Cephalopelvic Disproportion (CPD): fetus is too large to fit through the birth canal or the mother's pelvis is too small to accommodate the fetus

- ▸ Failure to Progress (FTP): cervix is not dilating or labor is not progressing, can be due to CPD

- Active Genital Herpes
- AIDS or HIV-positive status
- Previous cesarean, if the uterus has a vertical scar
- Maternal medical conditions: heart condition, severe high blood pressure, or some mothers with pre-eclampsia

Placental

- Placenta previa: low-lying placenta covering the cervix
- *Abruptio placenta*: placenta pulls away from the uterine wall
- Prior uterine surgery that has formed scar tissue, such as myomectomy-fibroid removal

Fetal

- Malpresentation-breech (buttocks or feet first), shoulder (coming out first)
- Fetal distress
- A fetal anomaly, such as hydrocephalus
- Multiples: twins, triplets depending on presentation
- Conjoined twins

Going Home

Don't rush your hospital stay because you are anxious to get home to your own bed. Insurance does not cover too many days of inpatient care, so take advantage of the full amount of time you are entitled to. In the hospital, you have nursing care, three meals a day, clean sheets, and pain medication whenever you need it.

Taking good care of yourself will enable you to heal faster so that you will be able to take care of your newborn. Let others help you. The less you do, the easier and quicker your recovery will be. The first week at home can be difficult. You may feel sore and uncomfortable. Remember, you are healing, and for the first 4 to 6 weeks, you should be waited on.

Sleep, or at least rest, when the baby is sleeping. Try not to do too much, even if you are tempted to. Your body will let you know soon enough if you are overdoing it. Conserve your energy. Follow your health care provider's instructions on dos and don'ts. Do not lift anything heavier than your newborn for 4 to 6 weeks after surgery.

Try to let your partner, family, and friends take care of everything. If you find that you do not have enough help, don't be afraid to ask for it. Most people don't really know what kind of help to offer you, so ask for specific things. Ask them to run an errand for you, bring over a hot meal, or have someone come over and watch the baby so you can take a shower and spend a few minutes by yourself. If you don't ask for help, you may not receive it. Most people will be happy to do things for you when they are asked.

If you don't have relatives who can help you, and your partner is not able to take off from work, you may want to consider hiring someone for the first few weeks. Postpartum doulas can be a tremendous help for the post-cesarean-birth new mother. They can help you with your newborn, and offer advice on newborn care and breast- or bottle-feeding. If you can afford it, hiring some help, such as a doula, can be both physically and psychologically nurturing for you and your newborn baby.

Your first week or two at home can be challenging. You are sore and uncomfortable and your hormones are fluctuating. You are experiencing all of the bodily changes and emotions of the postpartum period in addition to recuperating from major abdominal surgery. You may be exhausted, both emotionally and physically, plus you have a newborn baby to take care of. Keep yourself comfortable by trying a variety of positions for sitting or lying down can get you off to a good start. You can also try a variety of body pillows for feeding time to make yourself more comfortable. Try to sit on firm chairs, as you don't have the muscle strength yet to get up from a soft couch. It is good to get up and walk around as much as possible—this will help you to heal faster and ease discomfort from the gas pains you may be feeling, which can be intense after abdominal surgery.

If you experienced labor before your cesarean birth, you may have to deal with some vaginal swelling or hemorrhoids. Hemorrhoids could also be a result of the pregnancy itself. You can use ice packs for the swelling, and for the hemorrhoids, try some over-the-counter ointments or cream, such as Preparation H. Witch hazel pads can be very soothing for hemorrhoids as well. Bleeding and lochia discharge, as described in Chapter 2, can last up to 6 weeks. If you are bleeding very heavily (soaking more than a pad an hour), let your health care provider know.

Pain Control

You will probably be uncomfortable for the first few weeks. This is typical after major surgery. If your pain medication has been ordered every four hours, take it every four hours. Once you allow pain to build, it can become quite unbearable very quickly. When that happens, it is harder to get the pain under control. Take your next dose before the previous dose has had a chance to wear off. You may be fooled into thinking that you don't need the next dose, but pain can be unpredictable. Do yourself a favor and take your medicine when you are due for it, even if the pain feels as though it is not that bad at the time. Pain relief is essential to your recovery. Don't be stingy with your medication. Relief from pain will allow you to move around, and you need to do this for faster recovery. Moving your body will help you to get into more comfortable positions for breastfeeding or bottle-feeding and will help you bond with your newborn. There is no need for unnecessary suffering. You will not get addicted if you take narcotic pain medication for 2 to 3 weeks. After that time you can switch to an over-the-counter pain reliever, like acetaminophen or ibuprofen.

Staying on top of your pain can also reduce the stress of the surgery, which may affect your milk supply. Side effects of narcotic pain medications are drowsiness, nausea, and constipation, so while you are on it, make sure you are taking a stool softener or eating a lot of fiber. If you feel drowsy from the narcotic pain medication, be careful not to take it when you are alone with the baby. If you are still in the hospital and taking pain medication, and are alone with the baby, be sure to ring your for your nurse so she can take the baby from you. A very small amount of pain medication crosses into the breast milk. You can take your pain medicine immediately before you breastfeed so as not to allow the medication to get into the milk, and you will be comfortable while you nurse. Remember, you will only be taking the narcotics on a temporary basis, and your newborn will not be seriously affected by it.

Comfort While Recovering

You can try a post-pregnancy support belt for extra comfort while you are recovering. These belts can offer you support, which can make getting in and out of bed easier. They can also help to decrease swelling, reduce pain, promote healing, and protect your incision. These belts are available on Amazon.com and in most baby superstores.

DO...

- Rest and take good care of yourself.
- Eat small healthy meals and snacks throughout the day.
- Drink a lot of fluids, especially water.
- Spend as much time with your newborn as possible, apply skin-to skin as often as you can (except if you are taking pain medications and you are alone).
- Give yourself a break, and time to recover.
- Accept offers of home-cooked meals.
- Bring in healthy takeout regularly for at least a month.

DON'T...

- Lift anything heavier than your newborn.
- Drive for 4 to 6 weeks.
- Have sex until your 6-week checkup.
- Worry about keeping the house clean and cooking meals.
- Overdo it. It will set you back. Your body will let you know you are overdoing it.
- Have high expectations for yourself for the first 6 weeks.
- Feel anger, resentful, or guilty for not having had a vaginal birth. Labor and birth are unpredictable and this was the safest option for you and your baby.

Cesarean Scars

Focus on gaining strength and taking good care of your incision so it can heal faster. Your incision should be healing well and not be causing you too much discomfort. Your incision may feel numb, as the nerves in the skin were cut. Sensation in this area may not come back for up to a year.

There are different types of incisions that are used to perform a cesarean birth. The most common are the vertical midline and pfannenstiel. These incisions include the abdominal incision and the uterine incision. A vertical midline (classical) incision is rare today and is used only if the mother has had previous surgery and developed scar tissue. It is also performed in a dire emergency, as this type of incision takes less time to deliver the fetus. The incision runs from the belly button down to the pubis, and the incision on the uterus is the same. With this type of uterine scar, a Vaginal Birth After Cesarean (VBAC) is contraindicated since it can cause rupture of the uterine scar and uterus (Bonanno, Clausing, & Berkowitz, 2011).

Pfannenstiel (horizontal or bikini cut) is the most common type of incision. This incision is made horizontally across the lower abdomen, just above the pubis. The incision is the same for the uterus, just over the cervix. This part of the uterus does not experience contractions very

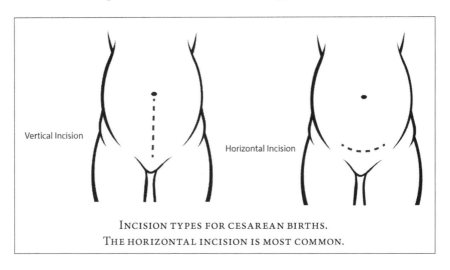

Vertical Incision

Horizontal Incision

INCISION TYPES FOR CESAREAN BIRTHS.
THE HORIZONTAL INCISION IS MOST COMMON.

strongly. It is also a smaller incision and less likely to rupture during labor. Women who have had these types of cesarean birth incisions have had success with VBACs. This type of incision also involves less risk, less blood loss, decreased incidence of infection, and fewer gastrointestinal complications.

Sometimes the incision on the skin and the uterus are different, due to the decision of the health care provider. A skin incision can be horizontal and the uterine incision can be vertical, or the skin incision is vertical, and the uterine incision is horizontal. Don't assume that if you had a vertical cut on your skin, that the uterine incision is also vertical, or vice versa. If the uterine incision is vertical, it is unlikely that you will be able to attempt a VBAC.

If you had a vertical incision, it will take longer to heal. A vertical incision on the uterus may have been necessary for certain reasons, such as a large baby or the type of position the baby was in. The muscles in the uterus will never be as strong as in a low transverse incision. The muscles will not have the strength to push the baby out during a vaginal delivery. This is one reason you would not be a candidate for VBAC.

During healing, it is important to keep the incision clean and dry. If you had stitches, they will most likely dissolve, and the internal stitches will dissolve as well. Always wash your hands before touching the incision. It will be sore and itchy for a week or two. Warmth, red streaks, bleeding, pus, or oozing are all warning signs of infection, so please call your health care provider immediately if any of these are present.

Gas Pains

Gas pains can be quite intense. This is caused by air that is trapped in the intestinal tract after surgery. Moving and walking will help to relieve these gas pains. Change positions frequently when in bed, or rock in a rocking chair. Eat light, easy-to-digest foods, such as soup, toast, and tea. The gas pain can sometimes travel to your shoulder and be quite uncomfortable. You can take simethicone (Gas-x, Mylicon, Mylanta gas) for the gas pains.

Constipation

Your first bowel movement can be uncomfortable, even if you didn't have an episiotomy. It may be hard to push since you need to use your abdominal muscles to do so, which are sore and weakened. In addition, due to the increase in blood loss, you may have been given iron supplements to prevent or treat anemia. Iron supplements, as well as narcotic pain relievers, can cause constipation. Surgery can also cause the bowels to become sluggish. Constipation can also lead to hemorrhoids. Getting on top of your constipation before it becomes too uncomfortable is important. Eating fiber-rich foods, such leafy green vegetables, fruit, dried fruit and prunes, raisins, bran muffins, and drinking a lot of fluids, can all help with constipation. Try drinking a full glass of real, pure prune juice, with the pulp, before going to bed. You should be able to have a bowel movement by morning. These foods will also help improve your iron levels. A sitz bath, stool softener, or laxative can help with constipation as well. Walking and moving around will also help get your system going (Graziano, Murphy, Braginsky, Horwitz, Kennedy, Burkett, & Kenton, 2014).

Splinting and Deep Breathing

When you cough, sneeze, laugh, or stand up from a sitting position, you need to splint your incision. This means to support your incision with your hands or with a pillow. You will need to ask for help, and arrange for help at home, especially if you have other children. If you have a toddler, this is extremely difficult, but you must remember not to lift your toddler. Don't try to do housework or cleaning—you need to let it go or wait until someone comes to help you. Deep breathing is very important to clear your lungs from the anesthesia and reduce postoperative respiratory problems.

Bathing and Showering

Keeping clean after a cesarean birth is important to prevent infection. You may be sweating a lot, especially during the night. This is normal after any type of delivery, and it is your body's way of getting rid of excess fluid that you had accumulated during your pregnancy. If you wake up in the middle of the night drenched in sweat, it is important for you to dry yourself off and change. This is only temporary and will stop in a few days. It is okay to shower whenever you want, although be careful not to scrub the incision site. Don't take a hot bath, as this can cause low blood pressure, and don't use oils, as they can irritate the incision. You may have staples, stitches, or steri-strips (adhesive strips), and these will be removed at the health care provider's discretion. You may experience itching around the incision site. This is normal. You can apply some Vitamin E to the area after any tape has been removed. When showering, make sure you don't feel dizzy or lightheaded either from the surgery or the pain medication before you get in the shower. Try to have someone there with you or just outside the door the first few times you shower, just in case.

Your Joints

The hormone relaxin was present in your body throughout your pregnancy, and is still present. Relaxin softened and loosened your cartilage, tendons, and joints during your pregnancy. These hormones allowed your pelvis to relax and open to allow the fetus to pass though the birth canal more easily. If you felt very floppy and clumsy during your pregnancy, this is the reason why. It can take a little while for your ligaments to retain their original position and you may still feel weak and floppy in the first few weeks (Sutton, 2009). Try not to strain doing household work, and don't start an exercise routine too soon, as you don't want to injure the ligaments until they had a chance to heal. Wait until your 6-week checkup and clear it with your health care provider before beginning any type of fitness routine.

Breastfeeding

Breastfeeding can be challenging for any new mother. For you, as a cesarean-birth new mother, breastfeeding can be a little bit trickier. Keeping your newborn skin-to-skin (see chapter on breastfeeding) is especially important for a successful start, and many hospitals are now encouraging skin-to-skin immediately after a cesarean birth (Elliot-Carter & Harper, 2012; Gouchon, Gregori, Picotto, Patrucco, Nangeroni, & Di Giulio, 2010; Kuyper, Vitta, & Dewey, 2014; Moran-Peters, Zauderer, Goldman, Baierlein, & Smith, 2014; Stone, Prater, & Spencer, 2014). Skin-to-skin contact is where you and your newborn are put together with nothing in between but your bare skin (and a diaper for your newborn, just in case). Use caution when applying skin-to-skin by making sure that you are not flat on your back, and that you have someone with you while you are still recovering (Davanzo, De Cunto, Paviotti, Travan, Inglese, Brovedani, & Demarini, 2014; Ludington-Hoe & Morgan, 2014).

You can practice skin-to-skin contact as much as you want at home. It will help you heal faster and reduce your anxiety, pain, and discomfort. There are many benefits to your newborn, including temperature regulation, a feeling of calm, and helping him to latch on and breastfeed. Even if you are not breastfeeding, you can enjoy the benefits of skin-to-skin contact (Hoffman, Massett, & Sorber, 2014; Hung & Berg, 2011; Moran-Peters et al., 2014).

As a word of caution, despite all the wonderful benefits of skin-to-skin contact, you need to be aware of some safety measures. If you are sedated from a narcotic pain medication, or are very fatigued due to a difficult labor followed by a cesarean birth, please do not be alone with your newborn while practicing skin-to-skin. If you fall asleep and your newborn is face down on your body, it can lead to complications (Davanzo et al., 2014; Ludington-Hoe & Morgan, 2014).

Keep your newborn off your incision and abdominal area as much as possible in the beginning. There are many positions you can try to help make breastfeeding as comfortable as possible for you and your newborn. A laid-back position with your newborn draped off of your side or a football hold—sitting up, holding your newborn's head in your hand with his back on the length of your arm with his legs and feet tucked behind you, are good positions to try. Placing your newborn on a pillow will make this more comfortable. (See Chapter 4.)

If you like the cradle position, try cradling the newborn in your arms—you and your newborn should be belly-to-belly. He should never be craning his neck to the side to get to the nipple, which is uncomfortable and can impede breastfeeding. You can place your newborn on a pillow, with his body facing your breast. The pillow will cushion any type of pressure on your abdomen. Make yourself a breastfeeding corner in your home where it is quiet and you have everything you need already set up. Sit in a comfortable chair; a rocking chair is a wonderful way to breastfeed. Keeping yourself hydrated is very important so don't forget a tall glass or bottle of water!

When to call your health care provider:

▸ Heavy bleeding, more than one pad per hour

▸ Clots coming from the vagina

▸ Foul smelling lochia or discharge

▸ Pain in the incision area

▸ Fever, over 100 degrees F

▸ Pain or difficulty urinating, dark amber colored urine, burning, or urinating very small amounts

▸ Pain in the lower leg, or pain when you flex your ankles

▸ Chest pain, which can mean a blood clot in the lungs—call 911

(Taimur, Haq, Khan, Kabir, Rahman, Karim, & Salahuddin, 2013).

Common Complications

Uterine Infection

Uterine infection is the most common complication post-cesarean birth. If you were given a prescription for antibiotics at discharge from the hospital, make sure you take the full dose for the required amount of time, as this will help prevent further complications. If you did not receive antibiotics, or if antibiotics were not effective in preventing or fighting off an infection, it is possible to develop an infection within the layers of the uterus. Typically, this is seen within the first 24 to 48 hours, but you can develop an infection at any time during your recovery. Factors that would increase your risk prior to the surgery would include gestational diabetes or an emergency cesarean delivery.

Signs and Symptoms of Infection

- Fever
- Chills
- Achy, flu-like symptoms
- Shortness of breath
- Pain in the abdominal area or uterine tenderness
- Foul smelling lochia or vaginal discharge
- Change in the color or amount of urine

Treatment

Antibiotics are the standard course of treatment. If you have already taken antibiotics, you may require a different class of antibiotics or you may need to take the prescribed antibiotic for a longer period of time.

Wound Infection

It is possible to develop an infection at the incision site. Bacteria can invade the wound, either during surgery or afterwards, either by your own hands or someone examining you. Risk factors include previous incision, as the tissue is weaker and more susceptible to infection, and a BMI >30, as flaps of skin cover the site, causing moisture and more bacteria to grow. Intravenous antibiotics during the cesarean are sometimes given to prevent this type of infection. Symptoms may not appear until a few days after the surgery.

Signs and Symptoms

- Redness or pain at the site
- Edema
- Ecchymosis (discoloration, black and blue)
- Fever
- Chills, flu-like symptoms
- Bleeding, pus, or oozing from the site

▸ Asymmetry of the site: infection will cause one side to be swollen and larger than the other

Treatment

Blood or wound culture to determine the type of bacteria. The incision may need to be opened and drained if pus is involved. Antibiotics are given orally.

Increased Blood Loss (Hemorrhage)

Excessive blood loss can occur either during or after a cesarean birth. Bleeding can be under control after the surgery, but it can start up again later on. The most common reason would be a uterus that does not contract properly. A "boggy" or relaxed uterus that does not contract can lead to excessive blood loss. There are many reasons for the uterus to be boggy. You could have developed a blood clot, or small pieces of the placenta have remained in the uterus, which could make the uterus unable to clamp down and contract.

Risk Factors

An emergency cesarean birth, Pitocin induction, or uterine infection before, during, or after labor.

Signs and Symptoms

▸ Excessive bleeding, or soaking through more than one pad per hour

▸ Feeling weak and clammy (sign of decreased blood pressure), lightheaded, fainting

▸ Heartrate is increased; you can feel your heart pounding

▸ Swelling in the vaginal or perineal area (bleeding can be inside the tissues)

Treatment

Massaging the uterus a few times a day will help it to contract. This may be uncomfortable because it is so close to the incision. Breastfeeding can also help the uterus to contract. Low blood pressure is one of the first signs of hemorrhage or excessive blood loss. When you lose a lot of blood, you lose blood volume to push against the wall of the arteries, which causes your blood pressure to drop. You may begin to feel lightheaded, weak, or clammy. If you are still in the hospital, the head of the bed will be lowered, and you will be given IV fluids with electrolytes, as well as Pitocin to help the uterus to contract.

Blood Clots

Pregnancy hormones release chemicals that cause the blood to clot, and lying in bed for long periods of time can cause blood to pool and form a clot. A clot can develop up to six months after cesarean surgery. The risk is higher in cesarean births than in vaginal births.

Risk Factors

BMI >30, difficult surgery with excessive bleeding, uterine infections, and a history of blood clots. Clots can begin in the deep veins of the legs. However, if one travels to the lungs, it can block the pulmonary artery and cause serious problems—even death.

Signs and Symptoms

▸ Isolated pain in the lower legs

▸ Swelling or redness in the affected area

Prevention

To prevent clots, you need to move around as much as possible. You may be reluctant to do this because of discomfort, but it is important to move your body as best as you can. The more you move, the better you will feel. While you are in bed or in a chair, you can try to bend and flex your knees and legs, and rotate your ankles.

Treatment

Blood thinners, such as Heparin, to break up the clots, or Coumadin, will most likely be prescribed.

Reaction to Anesthesia

General anesthesia can cause nausea or vomiting. Epidural or spinal anesthesia can cause shivering or shaking. Post-surgery morphine, or duramorph, that kept you comfortable for the first 24 hours, can cause itching. This is not an allergic reaction, but a side effect. You can take Benadryl (an antihistamine) for the itching. An extremely rare complication is paralysis from nerve damage, or from a blood clot or infection at the site of epidural injection. Either one can cause a bad headache or back pain.

Injury or Infection of the Bladder

Your bladder is pushed aside, and usually a Foley catheter will flatten it out during the procedure. Although extremely rare, the bladder can be nicked during surgery, which can cause urine to leak out of the bladder and into the pelvis, which can cause a major infection. Having had a Foley catheter can also lead to a urinary tract infection.

Signs and Symptoms

- Low urine output

- Blood in the urine

- Pain or burning on urination

Treatment

Antibiotics will be prescribed

Create a Healing Environment:

- Do not lift anything heavier than your newborn.

- Ask for help from anyone who visits or calls.

- No cooking, cleaning, or laundry. Accept meals from visitors. Bring in takeout. Use an outside source for cleaning.

- Consider hiring a postpartum doula, or ask a family or friend member to help out.

- Set up a few changing stations around the house supplied with diapers, wipes, and everything else you need.

- Eat healthy, small, frequent meals, and drink a lot of fluids.

- Move around as much as you can, and increase your activity gradually.

Vaginal Birth After Cesarean (VBAC)

Once a cesarean, always a cesarean?

During the last century, this way of thinking was commonplace. Once a woman delivered by cesarean section, all her other children had to be delivered in the same manner. In addition to that, the number of subsequent pregnancies was limited as well (Wainer-Cohen & Estner, 1983). A vaginal birth after cesarean (VBAC) was not practiced due to the risk of uterine scar rupture, which can lead to complications for the mother and newborn (Bonanno et al., 2011).

In the 1980s and 1990s, health care professionals and advocates argued this rule and encouraged VBACs. Surgeons found that if the surgical incision on the uterus was low transverse and horizontal (bikini cut), there was less risk of the uterine scar opening or rupturing during labor. When the uterine scar is vertical, as in the classical incision, then there is a danger of the scar opening and rupturing. Research at that time supported VBACs as safe, and as the risks of cesarean births began more evident, the decision to support VBACs became more apparent (Eden, Denman, Emeis, McDonagh, Fu, Janik, & Guise, 2012; Guise, Denman, Emeis, Marshall, Walker, Fu, & McDonagh, 2010).

As all things tend to go in cycles, recently this pendulum has swung back the other way. Controversy regarding VBACs caused another jump in the cesarean section rate with some obstetricians viewing VBACs as risky, and many began to decline participation in them. There is much conflicting information in the literature, and the hope is for VBACs to make a comeback. A VBAC can be a safe alternative to a repeat cesarean birth. If the reason for your first cesarean doesn't apply to the second pregnancy (for example, breech, herpes outbreak, or fetal distress), then you may be a good candidate for a VBAC. The hospital is the safest place to attempt a VBAC in case of emergency, such as rupture of the scar.

The National Institutes of Health (NIH) developed a statement on VBACs in June of 2010. It was determined that a trial of labor is a reasonable option for women who have had a prior low, transverse, uterine incision (NIH.gov/2010/vbacstatement.htm). There is also a guide to understanding this statement, called A *Woman's Guide to VBAC: Navigating the NIH Consensus Recommendations*. This is a free online consumer resource that offers good advice regarding decision-making with specific risks and benefits of repeat cesarean versus VBAC. You can find this at: www.Lamaze.org or www.givingbirthwithconfidence.org. Type in "VBAC" to find the guide.

You can also try VBACfacts.com for useful information regarding VBACs. It is ultimately your decision, and finding a health care provider who will support this decision and has experience with VBACs is crucial. Researching and discussing it with professionals and loved ones will help you to make that decision.

Uterine Scar Rupture

What exactly is a uterine scar rupture?
What are the chances that this will
occur if I choose to VBAC? Is it dangerous?
How will it affect future pregnancies?

The word *rupture* sounds very frightening. It is actually a tearing, a separation of the edges of the previous incision from your prior cesarean birth. Another term that is used is *dehiscence*. A rupture of the scar in the uterus is very rare, but can be serious for the mother and newborn, and requires emergency surgical care. Scar tissue in your uterus will stretch and grow as the uterus grows with your next pregnancy. Sometimes, the tissue around the scar stretches thin enough to cause a window or a thinning. This will usually heal by itself. However, in rare circumstances (less than 1% of women), it will separate and open (Ahmadi, Siahbazi, & Akhbari, 2013).

Uterine rupture can also happen in women who did not have a previous cesarean birth. It can be due to weak uterine muscles, multiple pregnancies, inductions, sometimes the use of forceps if they are inserted very high up into the birth canal, or other surgical procedures on the uterus. If the uterus does rupture, the immediate response is an emergency cesarean. This is done very quickly in order to prevent the newborn or placenta from entering the abdomen. Uterine rupture can cause hemorrhage for the mother, and anoxia for the newborn, which can lead to neurological problems and, rarely, death. If the birth is attended at a hospital facility, and the response is rapid, these problems are extremely rare. Immediate measures are taken to repair the mother's uterus and to prevent excessive blood loss. Women who don't have successful VBACs do not necessarily have bad outcomes. However, they will end up needing a repeat cesarean section after their trial of labor has failed.

VBAC or Repeat Cesarean Birth? Making an Informed Decision

This is a very difficult decision as it impacts you, your unborn baby, and future pregnancies. Some health care providers will agree that a trial of labor is safe if the mother has had a low-transverse uterine incision, is carrying one fetus, the fetus is vertex, and there are no other risk factors. You need to educate yourself as best as you can regarding VBACs and repeat cesarean births, and develop an understanding of the risks and benefits. You must weigh your own personal concerns and values, so that you can make a decision that is best for you and your family (Lundgren, Begley, Gross, & Bondas, 2012).

You may have had a bad experience with your cesarean birth, or suffered either physical or psychological complications. You may feel as if you would heal emotionally from your first birthing experience if you could give birth vaginally, or at least attempt it. You may not have any household help, need to return to work sooner than planned, or have a toddler at home to take care of. The thought of having a repeat cesarean birth may be making you extremely anxious, and you may feel as though you will do anything to try to have a vaginal birth.

On the other hand, you may have had a previous miscarriage, still-birth, or a difficult time conceiving, and view your next baby as so precious that you are not willing to take even a tiny chance of a complication from a VBAC. Or you may have previously had a prolonged labor, pushed for hours, and still ended up with a cesarean birth, and do not want to go through that again. Or you may have a small child and live far from family, and would like to plan your birth so you can have everything in place. This way, you will have the help that you need at the right time, and you will not have to worry about who you can get to watch your child if you go into labor in the middle of the night.

This decision is a very individual one and no one can make it for you: it is for you and your partner to decide. There are different risks and benefits for each option, and you have to decide which is best for you and your family. There will be some women who experience complications with a repeat cesarean birth, and some who will experience complications with a VBAC. Complications from a VBAC include a failed trial of labor that could end up in a cesarean section that is an emergency. If this were the case you might end up with a uterine infection. Uterine rupture, although rare, is still a possibility. There is no way of knowing the outcome, and there is no right or wrong

Good Candidate for VBAC

- A uterine scar that is low transverse (horizontal)
- Spontaneous labor (not induction)
- No use of Pitocin or a prostaglandin to ripen the cervix
- At least 18 to 24 months since your previous cesarean birth
- No reoccurring reason for cesarean birth, such as breech, malpresentation (buttocks or shoulder first), multiples (twins, triplets, or more), fetal distress, active herpes lesions, placenta previa (placenta is lying very low in the uterus, next to or covering the cervix), or abruption (placenta peels away from the uterine wall before birth)
- Good labor support, partner, family member, or doula

Poor Candidate

- History of two or more previous cesarean births, even if you have a low-transverse uterine scar
- Previous vertical incision
- Multiples: twins, triplets, or more
- Over 40 weeks gestation
- Unknown scar or other uterine surgeries

answer. Nonetheless, the number of complications for either option is still very small. There is no way to predict the outcome, no matter which option you choose. For this reason, you have to make a decision that is right for you and your family.

Emotional Healing

The most important thing is that the baby and I are healthy, so why do I feel so broken?

You may have had a chance to have your newborn with you immediately after your birth. Or you may have had your newborn taken from you instantaneously after birth, to the nursery for cleanup and evaluation. It may have been a few hours before you were able to hold your newborn. Don't feel as if your attachment will be compromised. It will not. Bonding with your newborn is a long process, and takes weeks, months, and even years. There is no need to think you are a bad mother. There are some things you have no control over, and you did nothing to cause the situation.

If you are able to be with your newborn, try to hold him as much as possible, and practice skin to skin. This will help reduce a lot of your anxiety and stress, which in turn will reduce your pain and discomfort. It may take a while for your newborn to latch on, especially if you miss out on the first hour of breastfeeding skin-to-skin contact with your newborn. Breastfeeding and getting started on skin-to-skin contact as soon as you can will help that process. If you are too uncomfortable, or in too much pain, you can have your partner or family member do some of the cuddling until you are able to.

Nowadays, hospitals are moving towards mothers keeping their babies with them, and encouraging skin-to-skin contact immediately after birth. This method has been created to allow cesarean birth mothers to feel as if the birth was somewhat "natural." This method of providing immediate bonding for cesarean birth mothers has been found to decrease pain and anxiety in the mother, and maintain body temperature and decrease stress in the newborn. This allows for bonding, easier latching on, and a better breastfeeding experience (Moran-Peters et al., 2014). If you have had this wonderful opportunity, you can continue skin-to-skin in your hospital room, with supervision if you are on pain medications, and certainly when you return home.

Your emotional reactions and adjustment to your cesarean birth are very personal. Emotional reactions to a cesarean birth vary widely. You may recover quickly and accept the fact that you had a surgical birth and that you have a healthy baby. Or you may feel cheated out of a vaginal birth. You may experience some level of sadness, disappointment, anger, loss of self-esteem, guilt, and depression. Sometimes, depending on the whole birthing experience, you can develop post-traumatic stress disorder following childbirth. You will be so busy with your newborn's demands that you may not have the time to process your feelings right away. You may be obsessing about the birth, and need to talk about it with whoever will listen. Or your feelings may emerge at a later time. Sometimes processing the birth may not happen until your baby's first birthday, when you are reminded of the whole experience.

If you are experiencing trauma after childbirth, those symptoms include, nightmares, avoidance, feeling stressed by reminders of the birth, and feeling edgy and experiencing panic attacks. Often mothers and mental health care providers confuse these symptoms with postpartum depression, and there is much overlap (see the chart on next page).

Some women may feel happy that they had a healthy baby while also still feeling upset, confused, or angry about how the experience unfolded. You may have a lot of questions about why things transpired the way they did (Puia, 2013). If your cesarean birth was an emergency, or if you had general anesthesia, or were separated from your newborn afterwards, or if your newborn had to spend time in the Neonatal Intensive Care Unit (NICU), it may be more difficult for you to adapt.

If you felt somewhat in control of your birth, and understand why you had a cesarean, it will be easier for you to adapt. Family members may not understand your feelings, and may tell you that you should be happy that you had a healthy baby.

Symptoms of PTSD compared to PPD

Symptoms of PTSD following childbirth

- Patient perceives an event as traumatic.
- Sometimes experiences flashbacks of the event with vivid and sudden memories.
- Have nightmares of the event.
- Unable to recall an important aspect of the event.
- Has an exaggerated startle response, constantly living "on edge."
- Experiences hyperarousal, always being "on guard" (ever present).
- Hypervigilant, constantly looking for trouble or stressors.
- Avoids all reminders of the traumatic event.
- Experiences intense psychological stress at exposure to events that resemble or remind the patient of the trauma.
- Has physiologic reactivity on exposure to events resembling the traumatic event, such as panic attacks, sweating, and palpitations.
- May distrust some authority figures and medical facilities.

Symptoms of postpartum depression

Five or more depressive symptoms (including one of the first two listed) for most of the previous 2 weeks, including:

- Depressed mood, tearfulness, hopelessness, and feeling empty inside, with or without severe anxiety
- Loss of pleasure in either all or almost all daily activities
- Appetite and weight change; usually a drop in appetite and weight, but sometimes the opposite
- Sleep problems, even when the baby is sleeping
- Noticeable change in walking and talking; usually restlessness, but sometimes sluggishness
- Extreme fatigue or loss of energy
- Feelings of worthlessness or guilt, with no reasonable cause
- Difficulty concentrating and making decisions
- Thoughts about death or suicide; fleeting, frightening thoughts of harming the baby, which usually tend to be fearful thoughts, rather than urges to harm.

Source: Trauma and Birth Stress–PTSD After Childbirth. 2011. http://www. tabs.org.nz/. Used with permission. Source: Postpartum Depression Health Center. Postpartum Depression – Symptoms. 2010. http://www.webmd.com/depression/postpartum-depression/ postpartum-depression-symptoms. Used with permission.

It is important for you to find someone with whom you can relate to talk about your feelings or find a mental health care professional. Before you move on to have another baby, or think about a VBAC, if you choose to, you must process your feelings from this birth.

How to process your feelings:

- Talk to your partner or family members about how you feel.

- Find a support group and share your feelings with other mothers going through the same thing. This can be an online group as well.

- Journal about your birthing experience, writing down your feelings about how things went.

- Discuss your birthing events with your health care provider and ask questions regarding why things went the way they did.

- Speak to a mental health care provider—if you are having a very hard time with this, you may need therapy and/or medication management.

Resources

Birthrites
http://www.birthrites.org/

Breastfeeding basics
http://www.breastfeedingbasics.com/articles/breastfeeding-after-a-cesarean

Mothering magazine
www.mothering.com

Cares Inc: Cesarean awareness recovery education support
www.caresinc.com

Childbirth Connection
https://childbirthconnection.org/

VBAC: A woman-centered, evidence-based, resource
www.vbac.com

ICAN: International cesarean awareness network
www.ican-online.org

Giving Birth with Confidence: A Lamaze blog for real women sharing stories finding answers and supporting each other
www.givingbirthwithconfidence.org

Hand and heart doula
http://www.handandheartdoula.com/Doulas_and_C-Sections.html

La Leche League International
www.llli.org

Lost Mothers: Cesarean support group
https://www.facebook.com/LostMothersCesarean

Mama birth
http://mamabirth.blogspot.com/2013/07/home-birth-cesarean.html

Prevention and Treatment of Traumatic Birth-PATTCh
Pattch.org

Postpartum Progress
http://www.postpartumprogress.com/

Solace for Mothers
http://www.solaceformothers.org/

VBAC Facts
vbacfacts.com

PATTCh (Prevention and Treatment of Traumatic Childbirth)
http://pattch.org

Chapter 4
Post-Baby Breastfeeding

*"Is breastfeeding
better for my newborn?"*
"Is it hard to do?"
"Are there any benefits for me?"
*"I am still deciding. How do I
know it's right for me?"*

Breastfeeding Basics

Congratulations! I'm assuming that if you are reading this chapter, you have decided to breastfeed your baby. The journey you took through your pregnancy and childbirth does not end there. It can continue with breastfeeding your newborn. You may have started breastfeeding immediately after birth, either in the hospital, the birthing center, or your home, and it is going well. Or you may be having some difficulty, and are on the fence about continuing. Or you may not have begun to breastfeed, but now that you are home, you want to try. It is possible that you have been experiencing discomfort due to an episiotomy or cesarean birth, or your newborn may have been separated from you due to illness, or for observation. Hopefully, by reading this chapter, you will gain the confidence and desire to continue the miracle of pregnancy with breast-feeding your newborn.

The benefits of breastfeeding are many, not only for your newborn's health and wellness, but for your own as well. Each and every female mammal produces her own specific milk in order to feed her offspring who need it for growth and survival. As a mother, your milk is produced specifically for your newborn, and is the optimum nourishment for her.

Your milk contains live tissue, live antibacterial and antiviral cells, a variety of hormones, and essential fatty acids that all play a role in your newborn's health and wellness. It is truly the very best way to feed your baby, and it is the way that newborns were intended to be fed. It is considered to be the gold standard for infant feeding (American Academy of Pediatrics, 2012; Brenner & Buescher, 2011).

Years ago, there were very few alternatives to breastfeeding. If a woman could not breastfeed her newborn, a "wet nurse" was hired. These women typically fed multiple babies in the community. There were no alternatives, such as formula or bottles. Yet breastfeeding was not automatic. It was a skill that was learned through other women. Mothers, grandmothers, sisters, aunts, or cousins passed down information on how to breastfeed. Girls observed other women breastfeeding from a very young age. It took a village to support the new mother and guide her and her newborn in learning the skill of breastfeeding. In today's world, there are safer alternatives to breastfeeding than there have been in the past, and women have many choices, but there are still some risks involved with not breastfeeding.

Breastfeeding is truly a miracle, and it is an extension of your pregnancy; part of your fourth stage of labor. It can be challenging, and some women may have a hard time getting started. Your newborn has an innate ability to find the breast, latch, and feed. Mothers also have breastfeeding instincts, but you may be too nervous to trust them.

You just need to give it a little time and a lot of patience (To learn more about mothers' and babies' hardwiring to breastfeeding, visit Biological Nurturing: http://www.biologicalnurturing.com/pages/philosophy.html, 2012.)

Your milk supply will seem to come in all at once, but will adjust over time in response to your newborn's needs. It will not always be as demanding as it is in the beginning. Give it time and you will see that breastfeeding can be a wonderful experience, and you will be happy that you made the choice.

If you are on the fence about starting or continuing breastfeeding, try it for at least a month. While it can be challenging in the beginning, it does get easier once your milk supply is established. Before long, you and your newborn will get into a rhythm of your own. Even if you stop after a month, your newborn will have gotten many of the benefits of breastfeeding for her first month, and if you can continue for three months, even better. Six months of exclusive breastfeeding is ideal because your baby does not need anything else until that time. After six months, she can begin to eat other foods, and if you continue to breastfeed, your breast milk will keep on providing its protective immunity and nutrients (American Academy of Pediatrics, 2012; Jones, Ickes, Smith, Mduduzi, Chasekwa, Heidkamp, & Stoltzfus, 2013; Spatz, 2012; U.S. Department of Health and Human Services, 2011).

There is no best method, position, or system to breastfeed, but there are some techniques and tips that might make it easier and cause you less frustration. Every newborn is a unique individual, just as every mother is unique. Your breastfeeding technique and feeding pattern will be exclusive to you and your newborn. This chapter simply offers guidelines for you, with basic information and guidance.

Breastfeeding Benefits

According to the American Academy of Pediatrics (2012), breastfeeding is the best way to feed a newborn during her first year of life because of the many health benefits for both mothers and newborns. There is no formula that can reproduce all of the vitamins, minerals, and other nutrients important for your newborn that are naturally found in breast milk. Breast milk is living tissue and there is no formula that can duplicate it (Eidelman, Schanler, Johnston, Landers, Noble, Szucs, & Viehmann, 2012). No formula exists that can offer your newborn protection against infection, bacteria, protozoa, and viral pathogens (including upper respiratory, gastrointestinal, urinary tract viruses, and bacteria). Breast milk offers your newborn all of these advantages (Lawrence & Lawrence, 2010; Renfrew, McCormick, Wade, Quinn, & Dowswell, 2012).

Breastfeeding helps you and your newborn connect to each other, and helps both of you learn each other's cues. Breastfeeding is not just a method of feeding; it is a way of comforting your newborn when she is tired, fussy, gassy, or overstimulated. There is no feeding schedule when you breastfeed, and after the first initial six weeks, it can be simpler, easier, and faster than formula feeding (Mohrbacher & Kendall-Tackett, 2010). You don't have to wash and sterilize bottles, or mix formula in the middle of the night. You don't have to prepare anything when you leave the house. There is nothing better than cuddling a nursing newborn in the middle of the night. Breastfeeding also forces you to sit down and relax with a glass of water a few times a day, and has a calming effect on you. Breast milk is always available, you can never run out of it, it is always the right temperature, and you can never forget to take it with you when you are rushing out the door.

There is also a cost savings, as formula is expensive, has an expiration date, and doesn't change with your baby's needs. In contrast, breast milk's consistency changes to meet your newborn's needs. Your milk will change in composition, from day-to-day, feeding-to-feeding, and month-to-month, in accordance to her growth and development. It even changes from season-to-season. It is richer and more concentrated in the winter months, and thinner, more dilute (containing more water) in the hot, summer months. The contents will also change according to her growth. Breast milk is quite amazing!

Mother Benefits

- Helps uterus to contract
- May protect against breast, uterine, and ovarian cancer
- Lose baby weight faster (you burn 500 calories a day breastfeeding)
- Delayed return of menstrual cycle
- Decreased lifetime risk for hypertension and type II diabetes
- May lessen risk of hip fracture and osteoporosis later on
- Relaxation during your feedings
- Empowering for the mother by knowing that you are giving your newborn the best that there is
- No need to purchase formula

Baby Benefits

- Contains immunoglobulins, which protect against viruses and bacteria

- Contains the perfect amount of nutrients for her needs

- Contains easily digested sugars for fast brain growth

- Contains protein that is digested easily

- Lowers the risk of allergies

- Helps prevent ear infections, asthma, and gastrointestinal illnesses, such as diarrhea, lower respiratory tract infections, and type II diabetes

Build Your Village

As many trends tend to revolve in cycles, in the 1960s and 1970s, more women were opting for formula feeding. Women were returning to the workforce shortly after giving birth, and health care providers, at that time, believed that formula was better for babies. Recently, the pendulum has swung back again towards breastfeeding, as more research in the literature has been supporting breastfeeding, and benefits for mothers and babies have been revealed. Health care providers and maternity staff in hospitals are encouraging breastfeeding, and more support is being offered to new mothers. Even so, women today may not have the same supportive network as we did centuries ago. A village to help them to get started, along with encouragement to continue breastfeeding. In today's world, your "village" is the place where you birthed, your postpartum nurse, your lactation consultant, and your health care provider. You may also be fortunate to have the support of your partner, family members, or friends who have breastfed their babies.

Becoming a new mother in this day and age can be very isolating. Twenty-five to 50 years ago, many women were all having their babies around the same timeframe. Friends shared pregnancy and newborn experiences and supported each other. Grandmothers, and even great-grandmothers, were available to help, teach, and provide emotional and physical support for the new mother. Many young people tend to learn by observation. Watching and observing other women breastfeed in the community helped new mothers connect to what appears normal, what positions to use, and how to tell if breastfeeding is going well. Breast-feeding stories were shared, techniques were compared, and those who had such support felt loved, supported, and empowered. Breastfeeding may have come easier to women with support as they had someone to ask for help when challenging situations arose.

Today, women are developing their careers at different stages. High school and college friends are not all having babies around the same time. Your parents or in-laws may still be working, or have decided to do more traveling. They may have moved to a retirement community. As a result, you may find yourself lacking companionship and support. Whether or not you are planning on returning to work, or you are planning on being home for a while, it is to your advantage to build a supportive network for yourself. A postpartum doula can offer you breastfeeding support, or you may want to have a lactation consultant on board for general questions and concerns.

There are many breastfeeding support organizations that offer local meetings. Breastfeeding USA and Baby Café are examples of organi-zations that have scheduled meetings where you can get to know other breastfeeding mothers. Seeking out other breastfeeding mothers will help you to feel connected. Having other new mothers to discuss issues and concerns with and having others to ask questions will give you the support you need while you are adjusting. The hospital or birthing center where you gave birth may offer breastfeeding support groups or classes. You can also try and connect with other mothers from your prenatal classes.

A Virtual Village

Build your supportive team virtually. You are fortunate that in today's world. You really are never alone when you have the Internet. There is always someone a click away. Many breastfeeding organizations have online support group forums that you can join. There are Facebook groups for all kinds of breastfeeding topics, issues, or concerns. You can even connect with other mothers around the world, and in different time zones. This way, when you feel alone in the middle of the night, it is someone else's day! You can get answers to your questions and concerns without waiting for the morning. Seek out resources and build your social network, whether in person or online, and you will gain the confidence that you need to breastfeed your newborn for as long as you wish (Audelo, 2013).

How Breastfeeding Works

Your breasts are made up of milk producing glands, and within this glandular tissue are many milk ducts. The ducts branch off further into ductules, and at the end of each ductule is what looks like a cluster of grapes—these sacs are called alveoli. A cluster of alveoli is a lobule, and a cluster of lobules is a lobe. Each of your breasts contains about 20 lobes with one milk duct for each one. During pregnancy, your hormones caused these milk ducts to grow in number and size.

In Chapter 1, I spoke about oxytocin being the "love hormone." Now, you are also producing prolactin (*Lactin* is the Latin for "milk," *pro* is to increase. Therefore, prolactin means to increase milk), which controls the manufacture of your breast milk and is one of the "mothering hormones." This hormone further enhances your mothering, nesting, and commitment to nourishing and nurturing your newborn. Prolactin was produced as soon as your placenta was delivered. When your pregnancy hormone, progesterone, dropped dramatically, this sudden decline stimulated prolactin, which caused the cells of the mammary gland to stimulate milk production (Mohrbacher & Kendall-Tackett, 2010).

As your newborn begins to suck, nerves stimulated by this activity send signals from the nipple to the hypothalamus (part of the brain that connects your nervous system to your endocrine system) to further stimulate prolactin release. Other hormones will also come into play to support milk production. As your newborn continues to suck, oxytocin is released, causing the *letdown reflex*. The letdown reflex, also called the milk-ejection reflex (MER), allows your milk to be ejected into the ducts, which become wider in order to carry milk to the nipple. The ducts are like the roots of a tree carrying milk to the newborn through small holes in the nipple area: the areola. It may take a few seconds, or even minutes of sucking for this reflex to be initiated. Once breastfeeding is established, this reflex becomes automatic, and may even occur when you hear your newborn cry, or are just thinking about her. You may feel a tingling sensation, or warmth, as milk comes into your breast. In the beginning, you may also feel cramping (afterbirth pains) coming from your uterus. Your uterus will contract as a result of the hormone oxytocin, which is released during your newborn's sucking.

The Stages of Milk

The first substance your breasts will produce is called *colostrum*. It is a thick yellow substance that does not look like much, but is very beneficial to your newborn. It is made up of the perfect amount of protein, sugar, fat, water, vitamins and minerals, as well as your own antibodies, immune factors, and enzymes. It also works as a laxative so that your newborn can push out her first black, tarry bowel movement, known as *meconium* (Mohrbacher & Kendall-Tackett, 2010). Colostrum is created during your pregnancy, and continues for the first 2 to 4 days after birth. It is very easy for your newborn to digest, gives her enough nutrition, and eases her into what is called transitional breast milk, which comes in on the third or fourth postpartum day (mature breast milk will not be produced until the 10th day). You may question whether or not your newborn is getting any nourishment. This is a natural process, and your newborn does *not* need anything else. Your newborn's stomach is the size of a shooter marble, and she only needs one ounce of colostrum for the first 24 hours.

Skin-to-Skin Contact and Breastfeeding

Your Amazing Newborn

Baby mammals have a natural habitat, which means home. The mother's body is the newborn's habitat. Skin-to-skin contact is a trait that is unique to mammals where the newborn is transitioning from the womb to outside life while still remaining safe, secure, and warm, nuzzled next to her mother's body. This is an innate behavior that is seen in all mammals after birth. All newborns have a strong sense of smell and respond to touch. Your newborn will smell your breast milk and start searching for it. After birth, when she is placed skin-to-skin with you, she will begin to move towards your breast in order to locate it and attach herself to your nipple for her first feeding. This is known as "the breast crawl" (Henderson, 2011). This process is all part of the miracle of pregnancy and birth.

The first hour after birth is a very special time for mothers and newborns. Meeting your newborn for the first time after nine months of anticipation is a precious moment. For your newborn, meeting you for the first time, too, after being secure and warm in your womb for nine months, is a precious moment for her. Your baby needs to have that continuation of being close to you, feeling your warmth, and hearing your voice. Skin-to-skin contact within the first hour after birth has been found to promote a newborn's first feeding, and helps make beginning and continuing breastfeeding go a little bit smoother. There has been a considerable push in hospital and birthing facilities to promote skin-to-skin contact immediately after birth, and to encourage it throughout the hospital stay (Moore, Anderson, Bergman, & Dowswell, 2012; Moran-Peters et al., 2014). Mothers are also encouraged to continue skin-to-skin after returning home.

Skin-to-skin contact is a multi-sensory experience for a newborn that stimulates her brain development, digestive system, and stabilizes their heartrate and breathing. Skin-to-skin is very soothing, creating a calmer newborn with less crying and less stress; a calmer newborn will have an easier time latching on and breastfeeding. Skin-to-skin also regulates and maintains a newborn's body temperature, reducing cold stress and helping her to sleep better. Breastfeeding more efficiently enhances your milk supply. It also keeps you calmer and more relaxed, lowers your blood pressure, and reduces your postpartum bleeding. Skin to skin has also been found to increase wound healing and decrease pain, which is important for you if you had a cesarean birth. Oxytocin is released during skin to skin, triggering contractions of the muscles in the breasts. Skin-to-skin contact is now being initiated with cesarean section mothers promptly after birth to allow for immediate bonding, decreased pain and anxiety, and all of its other benefits.

How to Carry Out Skin-to-Skin Contact

Your newborn should be completely naked except for a diaper (just in case) and a hat. Place your newborn on your bare chest, under your nightgown or robe, with her chest between your breasts, and her head under your chin. Her head should be turned to the side. Then, cover her with warm blankets, or you can use your nightgown or robe, making sure she is nice and toasty warm. You can stay like this for as long as you want, but try and remain this way for at least an hour. You will see that soon your newborn will begin to bob her head up and down, navigating herself towards your nipple. She is actually crawling towards your nipple. You can then help her to latch on and breastfeed. You can practice skin to skin as much as you want, and as long as you are able to. Every opportunity you have to practice skin to skin, take advantage of it. Skin-to-skin contact can also be practiced if you decide to bottle-feed so you can still receive all of the benefits of skin-to-skin, even if you choose not to breastfeed.

Starting to Breastfeed

Breastfeeding is a skill for both you and your newborn. Your newborn is born with a natural instinct to search for the nipple and latch on, all by herself. When your newborn's face is near your nipple, she will lift her head, open wide and begin to suck. Expect your newborn to fall asleep at the breast often, sometimes with the nipple in her mouth. She may suck, sleep, let go, wake up, and search for the nipple again. This is very normal, and this is how your milk supply becomes established. You can't over-feed your newborn—she will take from you what she needs, and your milk supply will build based on this need. Even though breastfeeding is a natural process, the two of you still need to practice how to do it, and learn each other's cues. As with any other activity, it takes practice, patience, and time. It will become easier as time goes by. Have confidence; you nourished your newborn all these months during your pregnancy without using supplements, and you can continue to nourish your newborn for as long as you wish.

Once your milk has arrived, and for the next two weeks, your breast-feeding habits will be settling into a rhythm. Your newborn will still be trying to get a mouthful of breast in and sucking hard to get the milk flowing. She will continue to suck, swallow, and pause, but once the milk starts to flow, there will be deeper swallows. She may still fall asleep at the nipple. Allow your newborn to finish with the first breast and let go before you offer the second breast. Let her take a little break, a burp, and then offer the other breast. Some newborns will only take one breast at a time, some will take both, and some will fall asleep, or nurse for a short duration, on the second breast. This is all perfectly fine, just be sure to offer your second breast first at the next feeding. Feel your breast to see which one is fuller. This will serve to remind you of where you left off.

If your newborn is still fussy soon after a feeding, you can always top her off with a few minutes of nursing. Don't let anyone tell you that your newborn is using you as a pacifier. It is your choice to use a pacifier, but offering your breast instead of a pacifier will keep her satisfied and help enhance your milk production.

What position is best to breastfeed?

There is no right or wrong breastfeeding position. The right position is the one that works.

Suzanne Colson

There are a variety of positions for breastfeeding. Most importantly, you should be relaxed, comfortable, and calm, or your newborn will sense your discomfort. Your back and arms should be supported if you are sitting up, and you might want to put your feet on a small stool to avoid strain on your lower back. You can use a pillow on your lap to support your arm or your baby. There are a variety of commercially prepared pillows available specifically for breast or bottle-feeding support, or just general comfort when holding your newborn (Boppy Pillow, My Best Friend pillow, Leachco Cuddl-U nursing pillow, NurSit nursing pillow, body pillow, nursing pillow, or a regular bed pillow). These can be helpful, but you don't always need them. You can purchase these pillows online, from any superstore, or baby store.

Some of these pillows wrap around your waist, so that your newborn does not need to rest on your arm. If you are lying down, your head, neck and arms should be supported as well. If you are reclining, you can arrange a pillow to support you behind your back. You should bring your newborn to you, and never lean over your newborn. You should be facing each other, belly to belly, with no gaps between you. She should not be twisting her neck to get to your breast.

Cradle Hold

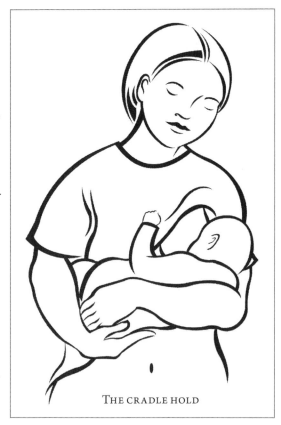

THE CRADLE HOLD

Sit comfortably. You can put your newborn on a pillow on your lap so you don't have to lean over. Place your newborn on your lap in a side lying position with her entire body facing you. Position your newborn so that her nose lines up with your nipple. Her lower arm should be tucked under your arm and breast with her legs wrapped around you with no gaps between her body and yours. Your baby's head should be resting on your arm in the crook of your elbow, while you support her body with the same arm. With your opposite hand, you can offer the breast.

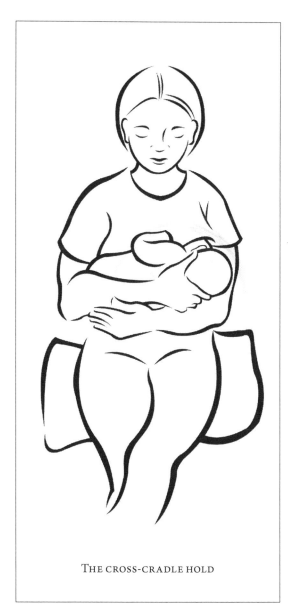

THE CROSS-CRADLE HOLD

Cross-Cradle Hold

Sit comfortably using pillows to raise your newborn's body to your breast level. Hold your newborn in the same position as the cradle hold, but with your opposite arm. Your newborn's neck and the bottom of her head is in your hand and your forearm is supporting her back. With the opposite hand, you can offer your breast.

Do not put your hand on the back of your baby's head as this will cause her to pull back. Many mothers prefer this position to the cradle hold because your hand on the back of the baby's neck gives you more control when you bring her to your breast.

Football Hold (Clutch Hold)

With your newborn by your side, put a pillow under her to raise her up and decrease weight on your arm. Your baby's head is in your hand, and her feet are towards your back. If you are feeding from your left breast, put her on the left side of your body; her buttocks should be resting on the pillow near your elbow. Turn your newborn slightly towards the side so she is facing your breast. Hold your newborn close to you with your left arm, tucked in well under your arm. Support her head with your left hand, and with your free hand, you can then offer your breast.

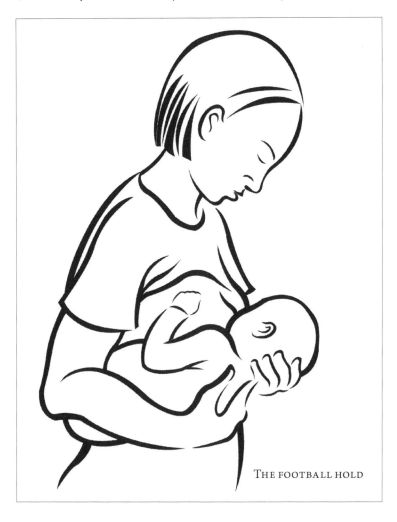

THE FOOTBALL HOLD

Sidelying Position

Rest comfortably lying on your side, using pillows to support your head and your back. You can also place a pillow between your bent knees to support your hips and take pressure off your abdomen if you've had a cesarean. Place your newborn on her side, close to your body, with her nose lined up with your nipple. You and your newborn should be facing each other. You can roll up a small receiving blanket or place a wedge behind her back, or you can support her back with your opposite arm. The sidelying position can be used for some mothers after a cesarean birth or discomfort from an episiotomy. If you had a cesarean birth, make sure your newborns feet are away from your incision, or he is loosely swaddled comfortably. It is an especially good position for middle-of-the-night feedings.

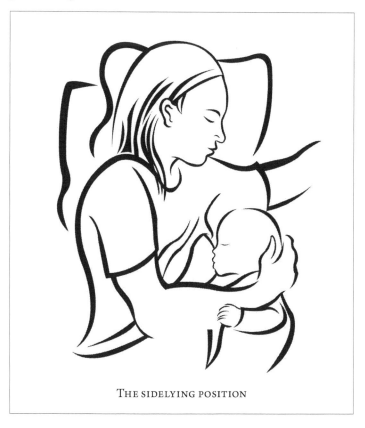

THE SIDELYING POSITION

Biological Nurturing/ Laid-back Breastfeeding

Suzanne Colson (2012) discussed Biological Nurturing (BN) as not just a feeding position, but a neurobehavioral approach to initiating and supporting breastfeeding. With laid-back breastfeeding, you lean back comfortably in a semi-reclining position and place your newborn on top of your chest top so that every part of the baby's body is facing and touching your body. Gravity holds your newborn in place, which frees up your hands. Your newborn is placed face down on your chest with her face near your breast. In this position, your newborn will use her natural reflexes in order to latch on. You don't have to hold your breast while doing laid-back breastfeeding, but you may decide to adjust it to make breastfeeding more comfortable. It can be helpful to watch a mother doing this rather than trying to read about it. You can see some examples at www.BiologicalNurturing.com.

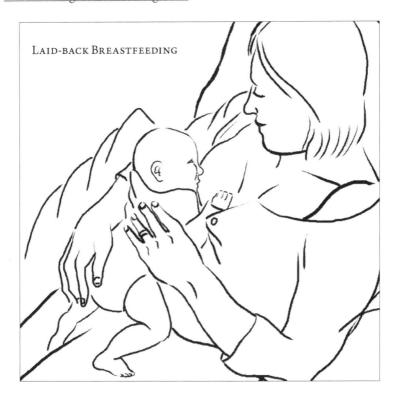

LAID-BACK BREASTFEEDING

Latching On: How Do I Know if My Newborn is in the Proper Position?

How your baby attaches to your breast is very important, not only for your newborn to receive nourishment, but also for you to avoid sore nipples, pain, or discomfort from breastfeeding. If you choose to feed in a sitting position, when you and your newborn are comfortable, you can then bring her toward your nipple. You can start by stimulating the "rooting reflex"—this is where you gently touch the side of your newborn's cheek with your finger or your nipple. This will stimulate your newborn to turn her head towards your nipple and open her mouth wide, like a yawn. You don't always need to do this. When your baby is showing early hunger cues, they will move towards your breast and try to latch on. Don't push the back of her head or thrust her into the breast, as this will cause her to pull back from the breast.

When your baby is latched well, your nipple will be far back in her mouth. If the nipple is not back far enough, she will suck only on your nipple, which will really hurt. Line up her nose to your nipple, place her chin on your breast, and you can simply "rock" her on to your breast. This will also allow her to smell your breast, and breast milk, and will then open her mouth wide for a good latch (To see an animated version of this, you can visit www.BreastfeedingMadeSimple.com.)

Once latched on properly, your newborn's chin and cheeks should be pressed up against your breast and her nose should be close to. You will begin to feel a pulling or a tugging sensation on your nipple. If you choose to feed your newborn in the laid-back position, she will bob over to your nipple and latch on herself.

Your feeding session will begin with a few short sucks, and then gradually, you will hear a low, deep sucking. You will then notice a rhythm of suck, swallow, pause, suck, swallow, and pause. Not every baby will show this exact rhythm; some will suck in bursts, and some will suck, suck, suck, and then swallow. There is no need to look at the time, but instead watch your newborn's feeding pattern and notice when she is not actively nursing anymore. She may either pull away from the nipple or fall asleep with your nipple in her mouth. When satisfied, your newborn will look totally relaxed and will have the same contented, floppy look of a "drunken sailor." Over time, the length of breastfeeding sessions may shorten as your baby gets quicker at removing milk from your breast. If you decide to take your newborn off your breast, don't just pop her off—rather, make sure you break the suction by gently inserting your pinky at the corner of her mouth before you remove her from the breast. Taking your newborn off the nipple without breaking suction can cause bruising or pain in the nipple.

When Latch and Sucking Are Going Well:

- Your baby has a mouthful of breast and a tight seal around the areola.

- There are deep sucking and swallowing sounds.

- You feel a pulling or tugging sensation.

- Your newborn's cheeks are not dimpled or puckered (middle of cheek caving in).

- You do not hear a smacking or clicking sound.

- You feel a tingling and pulling sensation in your breast, which indicates letdown. (Please note that some mothers do not feel this. No need to worry if the other things are going well.)

- There is no milk leaking from the corners of her mouth while she is feeding.

- Your breast begins to soften as your baby is feeding.

- Your baby detaches from your breast and appears sleepy and satiated (drunken sailor) at the end of a feeding.

Cue Feeding

How do I know she is getting enough?
How often do I feed her?

You may be surprised at how frequently your baby wants to nurse in the first 2 weeks. You can breastfeed as long and as often as she wants to. Your baby and your body are adjusting your supply. It takes time and patience, and it may seem that there is no clear pattern at first. In the first few weeks, you should be nursing at least eight times, probably more, in 24 hours (8 to 12 times per day), but those feedings may come in clusters. There may be times when your baby feeds every hour. Other times, she may go 3 hours before she feeds again. This will vary from day-to-day as your newborn grows. If your newborn is tired from birth, or if you received medications during labor that is making her sleepy, you will need to feed her 8 to 12 times a day, and this may mean waking her to feed in the first 2 weeks. The same if your baby was less than five pounds at birth, was born before 38 weeks gestation, has jaundice, or as indicated by your pediatric health care provider.

The length of time it takes your newborn to nurse also varies and may take longer in the first few weeks. Your newborn may fall asleep a lot at the breast, which could extend the feeding time to 45 minutes or an hour. If this should occur, make sure she is not too warm. You can also use breast compression and massage to ensure that she keeps eating and is getting milk that is higher in fat, as massaging the breast can increase the fat content in your milk. Newborns may also "cluster feed" (several feedings in a short amount of time) and then conk out and sleep for hours. Look for hunger cues (see below), and remember that crying is a late hunger sign. If you wait until your newborn starts to cry, it may be harder to get her to calm down and latch on properly.

The first 3 weeks of milk production are very important. Your newborn needs to consistently empty your breasts in order for your body to produce enough milk. Try to avoid any supplements of formula for at least the first 3 weeks, so that your milk supply can establish itself and adjust to your newborn's needs. Giving your newborn formula in the first 6 weeks may decrease your milk supply, as formula takes longer to digest than breast milk, so your baby may go longer between feedings. Emptying your breasts is your body's signal to make milk. If you stretch out the times between emptyings, your body will slow production.

Once your milk is established (can be anywhere from 3 to 12 weeks) the composition of your milk will change as well. You will be producing more watery milk in the beginning of your feeding. The high-fat milk is released several times during the feeding. Breast massage and compression also releases this higher-fat milk. Feeding length is typically 20 to 40 minutes. Some babies can drain the breast within 5 minutes. The best way to be sure your newborn is getting enough is by observing her dirty diapers, and by her behavior (acting happy, alert, and satisfied after feedings). She should have moist lips and mouth, and should be gaining weight steadily.

As a newborn, your baby's bowel movement starts off as a black tarry substance called *meconium*. This is known as stage one. At 2 to 3 days, your baby's bowel movements change to a yellow, seedy, thin liquid known as *transitional stool*: stage 2. This stage consists of a combination of meconium and fecal substance. Stage 3 is *breast milk stool*, which is where the stool is entirely fecal, and a pale yellow color, sometimes a pasty green. Breast milk stool is looser, more liquidy, and more frequent than those of formula-fed newborns, which is pasty, and more like a peanut butter texture, with a strong odor (Lowdermilk, Perry, & Cashion, 2014).

How to Tell if Your Baby is Hungry

Watch for hunger cues:

- Rooting (turning her head to face your nipple)
- Sucking hand and fist
- Moving head from side to side
- Opens mouth in response to touch
- Very alert, eyes wide open
- Restless, fidgety
- Smacking lips together
- Nuzzling against you

Remember, crying is a late hunger sign!

How to Tell if Your Baby is Getting Enough to Eat

- Audible swallowing
- 3-4 stools per day
- Steady weight gain
- Satisfied and relaxed after nursing
- Growing in length, good color, firm skin

Common Challenging Situations

Breastfeeding after Cesarean

If you had a cesarean birth, the time when your milk supply becomes more abundant may be delayed compared to women who have had a vaginal birth. You are recovering from surgery and will have some discomfort initially. It is important to keep your newborn off of your abdomen. If you are uncomfortable sitting upright, try the sidelying or laid-back position with your baby's feet off to your side. If you are comfortable sitting up, you can try the football hold or the cradle hold with your newborn on a pillow. You can certainly practice skin-to-skin contact as much as you like.

Flat or Inverted Nipples

Some women are born with flat or inverted nipples. Flat nipples will not protrude or become erect when stimulated or cold. This is usually not a problem for breastfeeding. You can to roll your nipple with your thumb and forefinger right before your baby latches so she will have something to grab on to. Inverted nipples retreat completely inward and can be coaxed out with nipple rolling or a shield. A good deep latch will help to draw out the nipple. A breast shell worn over the nipple can be helpful in pulling out the areola and stretching out the nipple. You can also try a supple cup, which you can purchase online, and can help evert your nipple.

Some mothers with flat nipples have found that nipple shields are helpful. Nipple shields are commonly used to cover the mother's nipple and areola, providing an artificial nipple for the newborn to use for a better latch. If you are having difficulty, it is a good idea to contact a lactation consultant, to give you an appropriately sized shield and show you how to use it. They may also evaluate your latch and help you make adjustments as necessary.

Sore Nipples

Some new mothers experience sore nipples in the first couple of weeks of breastfeeding. This is fairly common, and is usually a short-term problem. This can be due to a latch that is too shallow due to positioning or anatomical limitation in the baby's mouth (e.g., tongue tie), infection, or other cause.

There are several remedies for nipple pain that you can try:

- Make sure your newborn has a deep latch, so that the nipple is far back in the baby's mouth. If possible, see a lactation consultant for an evaluation.

- Be alert for signs of infection, such as fever, chills, flu-like symptoms, or red streaks. If you suspect an infection, contact your health care provider immediately.

While You Are Waiting for Your Nipple Pain to Heal

Once the original problem is addressed, you can try these comfort measures while your nipples heal.

- Offer your least sore nipple first, as a newborn's suck will be more vigorous the first few minutes of a feeding.

- Alternate breastfeeding positions at each feeding. Changing positions will force the baby to suck on different areas of the nipple, alternating pressure on the area of your nipple that is sore.

- Express some colostrum or milk and apply it around the nipple area that is sore or cracked. There are healing properties in colostrum and breast milk. This can be helpful unless there is an infection.

- Wash sore or cracked nipples with warm water, then air or gently pat dry. A gentle soap may be used a couple of times a day to prevent infection while the wound heals.

- Keep nipples dry in between feedings.

- Apply cool, moist compresses.

- You can try wearing a breast shell under your shirt, which will push the fabric off your sore nipples allowing them to air dry.

- Ultra-pure lanolin, such as Lansinoh, allows the wound to heal, as well as helping to prevent further cracking. This can be very soothing and protects cracked and damaged nipples. It is safe for mothers and babies.

▸ Hydrogel pads, such as Ameda Comfort-Gel Hydrogel Pads, or Lansinoh Soothies Gel Pads, provide soothing relief and encourage healing of sore, cracked nipples. They can also be worn discreetly under your clothes.

▸ If all else fails and your nipples are extremely uncomfortable, you can try pumping milk, using a hospital-grade pump, and feeding it to your newborn in a bottle or a cup for a little while until your nipples heal. Make sure that you are using the pump properly and the flanges (breast shields) that come with the pump fit your nipples properly. If they are too small they can actually cause sore nipples or add more trauma to already sore nipples.

Folk remedies, such as applying dried tea bags, and drying the nipple with a hairdryer, are not advised.

Contact a lactation consultant if you do not have relief from any of the above remedies in a day or so.

Engorgement

On your 3rd to 5th postpartum day, your body will experience a surge in milk volume and a change in the composition of your milk. This is sometimes referred to as your "milk coming in." You will experience a sense of fullness in your breasts, and they will become firmer and heavier. What is happening is that your milk is transitioning to full milk production. This is a normal process. Your newborn will feed differently, and you may hear more gulping sounds as she tries to keep up with the milk (Mohrbacher & Kendall-Tackett, 2010).

Your body is capable of producing more milk than your newborn needs. Milk production works on a supply-and-demand system. In order to increase milk production, your breasts need to be stimulated by emptying them. Initially, your body does not know how much milk your newborn needs, or how many babies you have birthed and need to produce milk for. Your breasts may look large and swollen at this point.

Don't be alarmed; as soon as your supply-and-demand process is regulated according to your newborn's needs, and your milk supply and your newborn are in a good rhythm, the swelling will calm down, and your breast size will most likely go back to the size they were during your pregnancy. This adjustment will usually take about 2 weeks, so hang in there!

Engorgement is different than the normal swelling and fullness you will feel after your milk comes in. Both breasts will begin to feel very hard, tight, and sore. Even the skin will look taut and shiny. Your breasts become so full that your nipple and areola are stretched to the point that your newborn cannot latch on. Some women feel the engorgement up into their armpits. This happens when your breasts overfill with excess fluid that blocks the milk from coming out. You need to express some of the milk. Don't be afraid that you will produce too much if you pump. Your body will adjust, but at this point you need to get some of that fluid out of your breast so your newborn can continue to latch on. Try to bring the swelling down with the use of cold compresses. You can also use a technique called reverse pressure softening (RPS) to gently push some of the fluid back up into the breast, softening the areola so the baby can latch. RPS can be very helpful in the first few weeks of breastfeeding. You may have received IV fluids during labor and postpartum, or have experienced general swelling and fluid retention which is common afterbirth. These symptoms can add to the discomforts of engorgement. RPS uses a gentle pressure at the bottom part of the nipple to gently push some of that fluid up into the top part of the breast. Using your fingertips around the areola, gently press back towards your chest wall. You can perform RPS yourself or with the help of the lactation consultant or health care provider. You can do this for a few feedings until you see your breasts become soft again and you don't have any more discomfort (Cotterman, 2004). (Check YouTube for videos demonstrating this.)

If you are very uncomfortable, try some cold packs for a short amount of time, or cool cabbage leaves. Breast massage before and during feedings can also help relieve engorgement. You can also take ibuprofen for the swelling and pain. Drink a lot of fluids, especially water, and wear a good support bra. Engorgement will typically last between 24 to 48 hours. Contact a lactation consultant or your health care provider if the engorgement is severe, or you have questions or concerns.

Plugged Milk Duct

The causes of a plugged milk duct are not well known, but several factors lead up to it. If you are a breastfeeding mother who has a good milk supply, but your baby is not sufficiently draining each breast, you can end up with a plugged milk duct. This is typically seen when a feeding is missed, your newborn sleeps a few extra hours, or sleeps through the night for the first time. Sometimes a too tight bra, poor nutrition, inadequate fluids, or stress can contribute to a plugged milk duct. Symptoms typically include pain or tenderness in one particular area of the breast, a reddened area on the breast, and/or heat arising from the reddened area. Treatment is to continue to breastfeed frequently, as this will help to draw out the plugged milk duct, as you keep the milk flowing. You can also apply a warm compress to the area, or soak the affected area in a bath or a basin of water. Medication or antibiotics are usually not necessary at this point, unless you develop mastitis.

Mastitis

Mastitis is a bacterial infection that does not cause harm to the breast-feeding newborn. With mastitis, you may start out feeling the same symptoms as you would with a plugged milk duct: a hot, reddened area, or pain in one particular area of the breast. In addition, you may also experience flu-like symptoms, such as fever, chills, fatigue, headaches, and muscle aches. The infection is usually limited to only one breast. The cause for mastitis is frequently a bacteria called *staphylococcus aureus.* You are vulnerable to mastitis when you are stressed, fatigued, or have nipple trauma.

The treatment for mastitis is to continue to breastfeed! It is a misconception that your newborn can get the infection from you through your breast milk. By breastfeeding frequently on that side (while not ignoring the other side, because you don't want the same thing to happen to your other breast) you will actually help draw out the infection, and milk will pull through and dislodge the clogged milk duct where the infection formed. Apply moist heat, massage the area very gently, drink a lot of fluids, get bed rest, and take acetaminophen (Tylenol) or ibuprofen (Motrin, Advil) for the fever and/or any discomfort or pain you are having. Wash your hands often with soap and water, use hand sanitizer, and be careful not to spread the infection. You can usually fight this on your own with proper rest and following the above recommendations if you don't have symptoms of infection. However, you should contact your lactation consultant or health care provider if symptoms don't subside or worsen in a day or two, in which case you will most likely need an antibiotic. A very small percentage of cases of mastitis develop into a breast abscess. This is a collection of pus inside the duct and must be drained by your health care provider with a small needle under ultrasound surveillance. Don't hesitate to get help for this, as some women may actually need minor surgery for this problem.

Breast and Nipple Rashes

Some breastfeeding mothers can develop a breast rash or lesion in the nipple area, such as eczema. This is an irritation of the skin that can cause burning, pain, or itching. Topical medication is usually the treatment for this, but be sure to wipe any ointment off before putting your newborn to your breast.

Candidiasis (thrush) is common in the breastfeeding mother. Persistent sore nipples, burning and/or itching can sometimes be a result of candidiasis. *Candida* is a fungal infection that is caused by yeast, and thrives in warm moist areas, such as the newborn's mouth or the mother's nipple. In addition to pain, you may have inflammation of the nipples and areola. Your newborn may have a diaper rash, and her mouth may have white patches and redness. She may also be fussy and refuse the breast. Candidiasis spreads quickly and can be passed back and forth from mother to newborn. You will need to see your health care provider for treatment with antifungal medications. This treatment should include yourself, your newborn, and your partner.

Medications and Breastfeeding

Health care providers follow the guidelines that are made available by the Food and Drug Administration (FDA), which has set up a letter grading system to help with decisions about prescribing medications to pregnant and lactating women. Medications are given a rating of A, B, C, D, or X, with A being the safest, and X being extremely dangerous (Briggs, Freeman, & Yaffe, 2012). If you are taking a medication, or are contemplating taking medication, it is best to discuss this with your pediatrician. There are many books regarding medication and breastfeeding (see below). There are also experts in lactational pharmacology who offer information on the safety of medication use while breastfeeding. Organizations, such as the InfantRisk Center or Lactmed, provide evidence-based information to new mothers, as well as health care providers, regarding the use of medications and other exposures during pregnancy and breastfeeding (see listing below). They also provide fact sheets and information on almost any medication, as well as herbal products, and vaccines.

Breastfeeding and the Workplace

I am retuning to work; how will I continue to breastfeed?

Many new mothers today are able to return to work and continue to breastfeed without too much stress due to all of the latest advances in breast pumps and storage equipment. Even so, returning to work with a new baby can still be challenging. You may enjoy your job but find that you miss your baby during the day. Breastfeeding is a good way to connect with your baby after a long day of separation. Your baby will also get sick less often if you continue to breastfeed, which is important for you, especially if your baby is in daycare (see resource list below). There is much more to say on this topic, therefore you might want to purchase a copy of Nancy Mohrbacher's, *Working and Breastfeeding Made Simple*. Also, check out the resources available at the U.S. Office of Women's Health and the Business Case for Breastfeeding.

Returning to Work:

- Arrange for childcare either at or near your place of work. You can go and visit with your baby and breastfeed during your lunch break.

- Invest in a professional grade pump and set aside time at work where you can pump in private. Store your milk in a refrigerator or a cooler.

- Wear nursing pads in case of leakage from your breasts.

- Keep up with your fluid intake throughout the day so you can feed your baby when you get home from work.

- Arrive to daycare or your sitter early so you can nurse before you leave your baby.

- Rest with your baby as much as possible when home.

Exclusive Pumpers

Can I just pump my milk and bottle-feed?

Some new mothers pump their milk and feed their newborn breast milk in a bottle. Although it is much more challenging than feeding from the breast, it is okay to do this. By pumping exclusively, you can produce enough milk to meet your newborn's needs for as long as you wish to offer him breast milk. Pumping frequently in the first few weeks is crucial in order to establish an abundant milk supply. Just remember that a baby is better at draining the breast and keeping the milk supply going compared to a breast pump. You will need to work harder at pumping in order for your milk supply to keep up with your baby's needs.

It is a good idea to rent or invest in a high quality hospital-grade double electric pump as they are better in many ways than hand-held or electric personal-use pumps. A single-user electric pump, such as a Pump In Style or Purely Yours, will work well for mothers who are pumping a few times a day after returning to work. However, they are not powerful enough to sustain the milk supply of an exclusively pumping mother. You will need to pump and drain your breasts as efficiently as possible. A hospital-grade pump is faster and more effective at emptying your breasts. Most hospital-grade pumps are double breasted, which will pump both breasts at the same time, thus cutting your pumping time in half. Some models can actually duplicate your newborn's sucking pattern, starting off with short fast pumps to stimulate the letdown reflex, and then becoming deeper and slower.

Most of the baby superstores have breast pump rentals, or you can find some additional resources at the end of this chapter. You will need to produce roughly 24 ounces a day for up to the first 6 months. Pump the amount of times that your newborn feeds within a 24-hour period during the day and at night (Mohrbacher, 2011). Make sure you completely drain both breasts, which will take anywhere from 10 to 20 minutes. Pump until the milk stops flowing, and then pump a minute or two longer.

Make sure the flanges fit onto your nipples correctly and that they are not too tight. If you do experience soreness in the nipple area, you can apply ultra-pure lanolin, such as Lansinoh (see below). If you feel as if your milk production is decreasing or you are pumping less milk, try pumping more often or for longer periods of time. If you are producing more than you need, you can always freeze your milk for later use. Having as many bottles of expressed milk as possible in the freezer will give you peace of mind and they will not go to waste (Mohrbacher, 2011).

Storing Pumped Breast Milk

- Room temperature: up to 6-8 hours.

- Insulated cooler: 24 hours (ice pack should be touching bottle at all times, try not to open and close bag).

- Refrigerator (not on the door): 5 days maximum, put bottle towards the back of the fridge.

- Freezer inside a refrigerator: 2 weeks.

- Freezer compartment with separate door: 3-6 months.

- Deep freezer: up to 6-12 months.

The Academy of Breastfeeding Medicine Protocol, A. B. M. (2010)

Keeping Your Milk Supply Going

- If you don't have one already, use a hospital-grade pump.

- Double pump both breasts at the same time as this can increase prolactin.

- Apply warm compresses before pumping.

- Relax when pumping, listen to music, read, or connect with your newborn.

Resources

Breastfeeding Online
http://www.breastfeedingonline.com/

Breastfeeding Resource Center
http://www.breastfeedingresource-center.org/

BreastfeedingMadeSimple.com
http://www.breastfeedingmadesimple.com

KellyMom: Evidence-based breastfeeding and parenting
http://www.KellyMom.com

La Leche League International
http://www.llli.org/nb/nbmarapr06p82.html

The Breastfeeding Mother's Guide to Making More Milk
http://makingmoremilk.com/

The Leaky Boob
http://theleakyboob.com/

NCSL National Conference of State Legislators
www.ncsl.org/IssuesResearch/Health/BreastfeedingLaws/tabid/14389/Default.aspx

The Adoptive Breastfeeding Resource Website
http://www.fourfriends.com/abrw/

Women and Infants
http://www.womenandinfants.org

Lansinoh: Breastfeeding and pumping products for mothers
https://www.lansinoh.com/about/lansinoh

Organization of Teratology Information Specialists (OTIS)
http://www.mothertobaby.org/

InfantRisk Center Texas Tech University Health Sciences Center
www.infantrisk.com

WomensHealth.gov: Office on women's health, U.S. Department of Health and Human Services
http://www.womenshealth.gov/pregnancy/

Working and Breastfeeding Made Simple by Nancy Mohrbacher
www.nancymohrbacher.com

Chapter 5
Post-Baby If Not Breastfeeding

"I have decided not to breastfeed. How do I dry up my milk?"
"What formula should I use?"
"What supplies do I need?"
"How often do I feed my newborn?"

Choosing to Bottle-Feed

The decision of how to feed your newborn is a very personal one for any new mother. Not all new mothers choose to, or are able to, breastfeed. Breastfeeding may or may not be right for you at this time, with this baby. Due to the stronger emphasis that has been put on breastfeeding in recent years, you may feel pressured, or even guilty if you bottle-feed. This chapter is written to support ways for you to bottle-feed successfully. There are many ways to bond with your newborn, no matter which way you feed him. Feeding your newborn is a time to cuddle, connect, and form an attachment to your baby (Labbok, 2008). Skin-to-skin contact is not limited to breastfeeding, and you can still practice skin-to-skin contact with your newborn in between or during feedings.

If you do decide to bottle-feed, you can still prepare your baby's food with the love and warmth that comes naturally when a new mother feeds her newborn. Make feeding time count by holding your baby skin-to-skin, holding him close to you during and after feedings, and becoming aware of his hunger cues. Make eye contact as much as possible, talk, coo, or sing to your baby during and after feedings. You and your baby can bond and attach while bottle-feeding.

Reasons Why You May Be Unable To Breastfeed

▸ You have T-cell leukemia virus type 1 (HTLV-1), which can be transmitted through breast milk.

▸ You have had surgery or trauma to the breasts where the ducts have been severed, such as breast reduction or enhancement, cancer, or tumor removal. Minor breast surgery, such as biopsy or removal of a lump, depending on how it was done, may also affect the ability to breastfeed if nerves around the areola have been cut.

▸ You have a medical illness that prevents you from nursing or pumping.

▸ You are taking medications that are contraindicated in breast-feeding, such as some chemotherapy radioactive agents.

▸ You are HIV positive and are living in a developed country.

▸ Your newborn is ill or premature and you don't/didn't have breast-feeding support.

▸ Your baby has galactosemia, a rare hereditary disorder where she cannot break down sugars in any milk, even breast milk.

▸ Your newborn has PKU (phenylketonuria)—you can breastfeed with supplementation with phenylalanine free formula.

(Odom, Li, Scanlon, Perrine, & Grummer-Strawn, 2013).

Formula-Feeding Fundamentals

In order to choose the right formula that is the best suited for your newborn, you may have to experiment with a few. While there are many different formulas on the market today, there are basically three types: modified-milk based, soy based, and elemental (which means that the fat, protein, and carbohydrate content is modified as in a lactose-free formula). These formulas also come prepared in four different forms:

▸ **Individually prepackaged and prepared bottles:** these are the most expensive, but very convenient. No refrigeration is necessary unless opened.

- ▸ **Ready to pour from a can:** also expensive, but no dilution necessary.

- ▸ **Condensed liquid:** you need to dilute with an equal amount of water; less expensive.

- ▸ **Powder:** you need to combine with water, but these are the least expensive (not sterile).

Individually prepackaged, or ready-to-feed formula is the easiest to use because it does not require any mixing, sterilization, or refrigeration. Although expensive, you may want to have a few bottles on hand to use when you will not have water available, or a babysitter will be feeding your newborn, and you don't want to worry about the sitter mixing formula improperly.

Formula concentrate is commercially sterile, but requires dilution with water. Be very careful: never give this to your newborn straight up, as it is twice the concentration of what you should be giving him.

Powdered formula, while the least expensive, is not sterile. If your newborn is very sensitive, has a compromised immune system, or needs sterile formula, this would not be a good choice for you. Powdered formula needs no refrigeration and is easy to take with you on trips. You can make up one bottle at a time, or several, but they must be used within 24 hours. You can warm them up for use by placing in a pot of warm water or letting warm water run over the bottle. Follow the directions on the can carefully. Since the powder is not sterile, it is very important that you wash your hands thoroughly and are careful to avoid contamination with germs. Make sure you mix the powder well to avoid clumping, but don't shake too vigorously, as it can create foam bubbles which can cause gas. Let the bottle sit for a few minutes to allow the bubbles to subside.

Whatever type of formula you choose, you need to make sure that you know the proper way to prepare and refrigerate your selected formula. Make sure you, and whoever will be feeding your newborn, are aware of the proper way to mix, reconstitute, refrigerate, and warm the bottle of formula for feeding time. Adding too little water can create problems with digestion, which can affect the kidneys and cause dehydration, and adding too much water can dilute the nutrients and calories that your newborn needs, and can lead to malnourishment. Ask your pediatric health care provider about using tap water for mixing. Some pediatric health care providers recommend all water be boiled for 1 to 2 minutes prior to mixing.

What Type Of Equipment Do I Need?

- ► At least 4-6 bottles and nipples
- ► A bottlebrush
- ► A measuring cup
- ► A plastic knife for leveling off powdered formula

Thoroughly cleaning all bottle-feeding equipment is very important, as milk can be a breeding ground for bacteria that can cause stomach problems for your newborn. Everything that comes into contact with your formula and bottle equipment needs to be cleaned. Check with your pediatric health care provider on whether or not they recommend sterilization. Wash all equipment inside and out with warm soapy water. With a bottlebrush, clean the bottom of the bottle and bottle rim, and turn the nipples inside and out, and scrub clean.

There are a variety of bottles and nipples available on the market. There are plastic, glass, or bottles with disposable bottle bags. Most are designed to minimize air intake while the newborn feeds. Nipples are made from rubber or silicone. If the family is sensitive to latex, you may choose to use the clear silicone nipples. There are also slow flow nipples for newborns that gulp too much air.

If your newborn is breastfed and you are using supplements or breast milk in a bottle, an easier transition from breast to bottle is a nipple that is not too firm. There is no one particular design that is best; the choice is by personal preference.

There is some concern about certain chemicals used in manufacturing baby bottles. Some research suggests that Bisphenol-A (BPA) can leak into the milk, and animal studies have shown that BPA can cause

Sanitary and Safe Formula Preparation

- Wash hands with soap and water before mixing formula, pumping, or bottle-feeding your newborn.

- Check the expiration date.

- Check how long you can safely store mixed formula.

- Never freeze formula.

- Wash the top of the formula can with soap and water before opening it.

- Make sure all bottles, nipples, and accessories are clean by either boiling in water, using microwave sterilization, or washing with warm soapy water using a bottle and nipple brush.

- Make sure you have the correct formula-to-water ratio for whichever type of formula preparation you are using.

- Check with your pediatric health care provider regarding your water supply and what type of water to use: different areas have different amounts of fluoride, which may not be beneficial to your newborn. If in doubt, you can always boil the water before using.

- Heat formula by placing the bottle in a bowl of warm water, or running warm tap water over the bottle for a few minutes.

- Some newborns prefer formula at room temperature and some prefer it a little warmer. Once formula is warmed it should be discarded after one hour.

- Never microwave formula, as different parts of the formula can heat up and burn your newborn's tongue and mouth.

- Any formula left over should be discarded within an hour (once your newborn's saliva comes into contact with the formula, bacteria can begin to grow). Freshly prepared, unused formula can remain at room temperature for two hours, 24 hours in the refrigerator for mixed powders, and 48 hours for liquid concentrate or ready-to-feed.

- Transport formula in a cooler with ice packs.

- Keep mixed formula bottles in the back of the refrigerator and not on the refrigerator door.

developmental, neural, and reproductive problems. Also avoid bottles made from polyvinyl chloride (PVC), which can contain lead. Many bottle companies advertise that they contain no BPA, PVC, lead, or phthalates. Read product labels before purchasing any bottle equipment.

How Often Do I Feed My Newborn? How Much?

The amount of formula needed by each newborn over a 24-hour period of time depends on the newborn's age and weight. Newborns are able to regulate their food intake according to his own needs, which can vary from day-to-day and week-to-week. He will express signs of hunger and satiety, and expect you to respond to his cues. Unless medically indicated (due to prematurity or illness), newborns should be bottle-fed on demand the same as you would with breastfeeding. Feed your newborn when they are hungry. (See information on early hunger signs in the previous chapter)

Your newborn will need to feed an average of 8 to 12 times within 24 hours. On average, this would be about 2 to 3 ounces of formula per feeding (every two to four hours) during the first few weeks. According to the American Academy of Pediatrics (AAP, 2015), your newborn will need to consume 2 and a half ounces per pound of body weight, per day. Therefore, an 8-pound newborn will need 2 ounces at a time, 10 times per day. Remember, this is an average guideline; don't hold to it too strictly, and feed him when hungry. This number will increase as your newborn continues to grow. Growth spurts will occur at approximately 10 days, 3 weeks, 6 weeks, 3 months, and 6 months. After 6 months, he will drink less because you will probably be introducing solid foods. It is always best to check with your pediatric health care provider regarding how much your baby should be getting each day depending on his weight (United States Department of Food and Agriculture [USDA], 2014).

Don't force your newborn to finish a bottle, and don't put him on a strict feeding schedule, or you may cause your newborn to be over- or underfed. Look for hunger and satiety cues. A healthy newborn will establish his own pattern according to individual growth requirements.

Let the baby set the pace for a feeding, which can take anywhere from 20 to 30 minutes. In the beginning, your infant may pause a few times, or snooze a little. When he lets go of the nipple or empties the bottle, it is time to take the bottle away. Always burp your newborn halfway, and then again after the bottle is finished. During a feeding, your newborn can develop an air bubble that can become trapped underneath the formula they are drinking, after which they can spit up all the formula on top of the air bubble. Bottle-fed newborns need more burping than breastfed newborns because the flow is faster and they tend to gulp more air, especially when hungry. If your newborn is leaking milk from the sides of his mouth, he may be getting the formula too quickly. Try using a slower-flow nipple.

Signs of Fullness

- ► Decreases sucking.
- ► Sealing his lips together.
- ► Pushes the nipple out with his tongue.
- ► Turns away from the bottle.

How Do I Know If He Is Getting Enough?

- ► Gaining weight.
- ► Looks relaxed and satisfied after a feeding.
- ► Has 6-8 wet diapers per day. Stool can vary in formula-fed newborn: he can have 1 or 2 per day, not have 1 for a few days, or have 5 in one day. Make sure your newborn is moving his bowels and that the stool is not too hard. Sometimes the iron in the formula can cause constipation.

Bottle-Feeding Your Newborn

DO...

▶ Wash hands with soap and water.

▶ Find a comfortable place to feed him, in a quiet spot like a rocking chair.

▶ Always hold your newborn when feeding, make sure you are relaxed and in a comfortable position.

▶ Use a feeding or body pillow for comfort.

▶ Sit in a comfortable chair with your arm supported.

▶ Position him in the crook of your arm at a 45-degree angle, and let him see your face.

▶ His head should be a little bit forward, higher than the rest of his body; the head should not be tilted back or lying flat.

▶ Stroke his cheek (rooting reflex) and your newborn will turn towards you and open his mouth.

▶ Keep him upright for at least 15 minutes, and try for a burp before putting to sleep.

▶ Tip the bottle so there is milk in the nipple, to avoid gas bubbles.

▶ Make sure the formula is not flowing too fast or too slow (if held upside down, the drops should follow each other closely and not make a stream).

▶ Interact while you feed; cuddle, coo, talk or sing to him.

DON'T...

▶ Prop a bottle. It can cause choking, overfeeding, ear infections, dental problems, and your newborn will lack human contact.

▶ Push or overfeed. Allow your baby to let you know when he is done feeding.

▶ Feed your newborn in a lying down position, in a car seat, carrier, stroller, crib, or infant seat.

Lactation Suppression

How Do I Dry Up My Breast Milk?

If you decide to bottle-feed your newborn, you will have to suppress your milk. Even though you will not have your newborn sucking and stimulating milk production, your milk may still come in on your second to fourth postpartum day. You will have colostrum in your breasts for the first day or two, and then your milk may fill your breasts; without the stimulation of a newborn sucking, this will become somewhat uncomfortable. There are some herbs that can help to decrease milk production. The spices sage and parsley have been shown to reduce milk supply. Peppermint has also been shown to decrease milk production and is sometimes used to treat engorgement (West & Marasco, 2009). Some medications to suppress milk production are not safe and are not used today. Sudafed (pseudophedrine) is typically used as a decongestant, and can help to dry up your milk supply under the guidance of your health care provider. Cabbage leaves can also be used to relieve engorgement while your milk supply decreases (Cole, 2012). Always speak to your health care provider before beginning any medication or herbal treatments for lactation suppression.

To be more comfortable while your milk supply decreases, try the following:

- Wear a good support bra 24 hours a day.
- Apply ice packs to your breasts to reduce engorgement.
- Use ibuprofen for the discomfort and inflammation.
- Don't stimulate the breasts, as this will increase your milk supply. If engorgement is very uncomfortable, you can express some milk for relief. Make sure you don't empty your breasts too much, just squeeze a little out for comfort.
- Cooled, green cabbage leaves are helpful for engorgement and maintaining comfort. Wash the leaves and apply to your breasts, leave them on until they wilt, and then apply the next cabbage leaf. Use as often as you wish until engorgement subsides.

Engorgement should resolve within 48 to 72 hours. However, it may take a few weeks, or even a month, for all of your milk to be gone.

In addition, "No more milk" tea by Earth Mama Angel Baby is a blend of herbs that suppresses milk supply. It contains sage, peppermint, and parsley. Drink up to three cups a day (West & Marasco, 2009).

Milk Sharing

There are a few grass-roots organizations that are advocating a concept known as "milk sharing." These non-profit organizations assist families who have chosen to share breast milk, by either donating their own, or receiving milk for their baby. There are many mothers that are willing to share their breast milk with women who cannot breastfeed their babies. These women feel that babies should be nourished with breast milk, whether or not their mothers are able to provide it. These networks offer global networking and communication between mothers who want their babies to receive breast milk. The basis for these global networks is to encourage babies around the world to receive human milk.

There is some controversy over safety issues regarding the use of milk sharing. It is very important that a mother who is considering milk sharing to be aware of the risks, precautions, and safety rules for doing so. Women who donate milk are encouraged to use full disclosure regarding medications, alcohol and drug usage, as well as any infectious or communicable diseases they may have had. It is wise to find a network where you can view these test results. The receiving mother herself can pasteurize the milk prior to giving it to her baby. There are several websites that advocate milk sharing and have a lot of information on the topic, such as Eats on Feets, Milk Share, and Human Milk 4 Human Babies (see below). These websites provide networking and information on this topic. If you are interested in milk sharing, it is very important that you make an informed decision and decide what is best for you and your baby.

In conclusion, be secure in your decision of how to feed your newborn. Choose a mode of infant feeding that best suits your personal circumstances. You are capable of making the best decision for your situation. Newborn babies thrive on love, attention, affection, and good basic care. You can give your newborn the security he needs to reach his full potential, no matter which way you decide to nourish your baby (Williams, Donaghue, & Kurz, 2013; Wirihana, & Barnard, 2012).

Resources

Ameda
http://www.ameda.com/

Baby Center
http://www.babycenter.com/0_how-to-buy-a-breast-pump_429.bc

Breast Pumps Direct
http://www.breastpumpsdirect.com/hospital_grade_breast_pumps_a/154.htm

Centers for Disease Control and Prevention
http://www.cdc.gov/breastfeeding/recommendations/handling_breast-milk.htm

Circle of Moms
http://www.circleofmoms.com/topics/bottle-feeding-moms

Eats on Feets
http://www.eatsonfeets.org/

Human Milk 4 Human Babies
http://hm4hb.net/

Lactation Connection
http://www.lactationconnection.com/Breast-Pump-Rentals-s/1834.htm

Lansinoh
https://www.lansinoh.com/products/hpa-lanolin

Medela
http://www.medelabreastfeedingus.com/products/category/breast-pumps

Milk Share
http://milkshare.birthingforlife.com/

The Upper Breast Side
http://www.upperbreastside.com/collections/nursing-pumps

Yummy Mummy
http://yummymummystore.com/pump-rental

Chapter 6
Post-Baby Diet and Nutrition

"My baby is born. Can I eat whatever I want, whenever I want now?"

As you must have discovered by now, pregnancy and childbirth have taken a lot out of you, both physically and mentally. This experience has also taken a lot out of your nutrient reserves. Although you had to be extremely careful about what you ate and drank during your pregnancy, you can relax a little about it now. You still need to eat well in order to replenish your nutrient stores, and to feel healthy and strong so that you can take good care of both yourself and your newborn. Whether you are breast- or bottle-feeding, you are going to need rest, energy, and endurance over the next 6 weeks and beyond. Replenishing your body and eating a healthy, well-balanced diet will help you to achieve this.

Eating Right

Eating healthy after childbirth is very important for you, as a new mother. More important than losing your baby weight is that you eat a healthy diet. By eating right, you will lose your pregnancy weight in a healthy manner. Eating right can provide you with what your body needs, to replenish your vitamin, mineral, and iron stores that were lost with your birth (Allen, 2012; Duggan, Srinivasan, Thomas, Samuel, Rajendran, Muthayya, & Kurpad, 2014). This is all easier said than done!

The "good" news is that the strong cravings or aversions that you may have had during your pregnancy will no longer trouble you. The "not so good" news is that with caring for your newborn 24/7, and being sleep deprived, you may not even have time to think about food, let alone prepare and eat it! By forgetting to, or not taking time to eat, you will deplete your energy and nutrient stores even more. Try to push yourself to eat well, even if you just graze throughout the day. You don't have to sit down to three square meals in order to receive the nutrition you need. Consume healthy foods and nutrients by snacking and nibbling on foods that you can easily store, keep available, and eat one-handed. Preparing foods ahead of time will help so you don't grab unhealthy snacks when you are hungry and in a hurry.

When you sit down to feed your newborn, take something to snack on for yourself, too. Keep a basket of healthy snacks next to your feeding chair. You can stash a banana, dried fruit, nuts, raisins, and other non-perishable snacks in your feeding corner. You can also put a snack bowl or bag in the refrigerator that you can bring with you when you sit down to feed the baby. Keep some cut up carrots, peppers, celery, cucumbers, apple, other fruit, or slices of cheese on hand in the fridge. Yogurts that you don't need two hands for, like ones you can squeeze or drink with a straw, are also good and easy to eat when your hands are full.

Keep it simple by choosing foods that are whole (foods that have not been processed or contain artificial ingredients) and healthy, but do not need too much preparation. Nutritious foods that are fast, easy, and simple include fresh fruit, raw vegetables, cheeses, yogurts, dried fruits (such as figs, dates, cranberries, and raisins), nuts, seeds (such as sunflower seeds), nut butters, cottage cheese, energy bars, or cereals. Try easy-to-prepare meals, such as sandwiches on whole-grain bread, finger foods (see the healthy snack list below), hummus, and whole grain crackers. For breakfast on the go, you can make a smoothie or protein shake. Use milk (skim, almond, soy, or coconut) or fruit juice, fruit, such as berries or frozen fruit, a banana, and some protein powder or a tablespoon of nut butter (such as peanut, almond, sunflower, or cashew), and you have a whole meal. A smoothie is perfect to sip on when you sit down to feed your newborn.

When friends and family ask what they can bring when they visit, don't be shy about asking them to bring healthy foods. Tell them you will appreciate meals that are simple to heat up, such as soups, a roasted or rotisserie chicken, beef stew, or whole-wheat pasta with fresh marinara sauce. You will need foods that are somewhat durable that you can freeze and re-heat. Ask them to stop at the supermarket and pick up a few items for you. Sometimes people want to help, but they don't know what to do or what you need, so don't be embarrassed to ask; if they want to visit, they should be happy to run an errand or two for you.

Food Guidelines

Be aware of these essential nutrients and some healthy options when planning your food intake:

Protein: high-quality, protein-rich foods, such as beans, legumes, tofu, nuts, seeds, lean meat, chicken, and fish

Carbohydrates: whole wheat, brown rice, millet, buckwheat, barley, oats, quinoa, and whole-wheat pasta

Vitamins/Minerals: fruits, vegetables, nuts, seeds, dairy, whole grains, supplements (prenatal vitamins, long-chain omega-3 fatty acids, Vitamin D, calcium)

Fats: Be aware of "good" versus "bad" fats. Nuts, seeds, avocado, fish, and healthy oils (such as olive and canola) are considered sources of good fat. Stay away from hydrogenated fats, as are found in margarine or shortening, fries, cookies, cakes, pastries, desserts, and chips, to name a few. Your body has to work harder to process these foods, making your body that is already depleted from pregnancy and birth even more deficient. Butter is a better option than margarine. If you avoid these foods, your excess weight will come off easily, your mood and emotions will be more stable, and you will sleep better.

The Breastfeeding Diet

Do I need to drink milk in order to make milk?

Cows don't drink milk and create plenty of it. Therefore, you don't necessarily need to drink milk in order to produce it! Nor does your diet need to be perfect for breastfeeding and keeping up your milk supply. Breast milk comes from your bloodstream, and no matter what foods you eat, your body will make the right amount of human milk protein. There are mothers living in developing countries who produce enough milk for their newborns. However, if you are deficient in nutrients, your newborn will get whatever you have left, leaving you even more deficient. You will become depleted of nutrients, such as calcium, DHA, and folic acid (Gartner, Morton, Lawrence, Naylor, O'Hare, Schanler, & Eidelman, 2005).

If you are breastfeeding, you will have to be a little bit more careful about what you put into your body in order to make sure that you keep up an adequate milk supply and give your newborn a healthy diet as well. Remember that you are burning more calories than you did when you were pregnant. You will be burning 500 calories per day while breastfeeding, as opposed to just 300 calories a day during your pregnancy. Therefore, you will need to eat a nutritious, healthy diet, plus 20% more! This is because your newborn is growing at a much faster rate than when she was a fetus, and is much more active than when she was in the womb (Neville, McKinley, Holmes, Spence, & Woodside, 2014). You need to eat 200 calories a day more than you were used to during your pregnancy. Examples of an extra 200 calories are fruit and a yogurt, or a peanut butter and jelly or turkey sandwich.

What do I need to limit or avoid?

There are some foods you may want to avoid altogether or consume in moderation.

Caffeine

Caffeine is not harmful in small amounts, as less than 1% of what you consume is transferred into your breast milk. However, 1 to 2 cups per day of a caffeinated beverage should be your maximum: 300 milligrams of caffeine (equivalent to 16 ounces of coffee) is the most you should consume. Be aware of caffeine in tea, soft drinks, energy drinks, and chocolate. Any more than the recommended amount can cause your newborn to become jittery and develop sleep problems. For you, excess caffeine can lead to anxiety and sleep problems as well.

Please don't smoke if you are breastfeeding. You will produce less milk and your newborn will not sleep well. Try a patch or nicotine gum for the duration of your breastfeeding. If those don't work, and you still need to smoke, don't do so around or near your newborn. Your car and house should be free from smoke. Be aware that there is an association between sudden infant death syndrome and tobacco exposure.

Alcohol

Alcohol does pass into breast milk. A small amount, such as one drink or a glass of wine is okay on occasion. You do not need to "pump and dump," as the alcohol does not remain in your milk, but it reabsorbed back into your body. Pumping also does not speed the process of getting rid of the alcohol in your breast milk. An occasional celebratory single, small, alcoholic drink is acceptable. Allow at least two hours to pass per drink before you breastfeed or pump. That way, your body will have as much time as possible to rid itself of the alcohol before the next feeding and less will reach your infant. Keep in mind that alcohol can inhibit milk production. Bottle-feeding mothers, you are not in the clear. An occasional drink is okay. However, alcohol and recreational drug use can impair your judgment and your ability to care for your newborn. No illicit drugs are safe for any new mother (Sachs, Frattarelli, Galinkin, Green, Johnson, Neville, & Van den Anker, 2013).

If your newborn is fussy, she may have some gas. Look into your diet and see if there is anything that might be increasing gassiness. Dairy products, eggs, peanuts, orange juice, wheat, tomatoes, and tomato sauces can also cause gas in the newborn. Experiment by eliminating some foods and see your newborn's reaction. Try and see the time of day that she is fussy, and if you can correlate it with anything you did or ate right before.

Some newborns just have a fussy time, or have "colic," no matter what you eat. By 3 months, babies will usually have outgrown this.

What about exercise?

Exercise does not have any negative effect on breastfeeding, but some babies may refuse the breast or become fussy after you exercise (Daley, Thomas, Cooper, Fitzpatrick, McDonald, Moore, & Deeks, 2012). Some practitioners are concerned that lactic acid in the milk may be a problem for babies following exercise. However, lactic acid only tends to build up in the milk after strenuous exercise (e.g., training for a marathon). There is no increase in lactic acid following light or moderate exercise, which is probably the most appropriate level for postpartum women (Quinn & Carey, 1999). Start slow and increase to moderate exercise, but not before six weeks. Wear a good, tight support bra when exercising, vigorous cardio can cause rubbing against your bra fabric, which can lead to mastitis.

Postpartum Weight Loss

My baby weighed 7.5 pounds, so how did I only lose 5 pounds?!
How long will it take to lose all of the baby weight?

You may be a little disappointed at the amount of weight you have lost immediately after birth. You may lose only a few pounds after birth, from the weight of the baby, the placenta, amniotic fluid, and blood. Your body is retaining fluids, and you are still losing the products of conception slowly through your lochia. You will be able to lose weight simply by shedding fluids and eating the right foods. Some new mothers lose weight quickly, but for others, it may happen a bit more slowly, depending on how much fluid you are retaining and your general metabolism. Don't compromise your own health, and your newborn's, to have the perfect body after a few months. Strive to be healthy while you eat right and exercise lightly. In the following weeks, you will lose excess water, then about 1 to 2 pounds per month for 4 to 6 months. This rate is different for everyone.

You may have heard that you lose weight faster when breast-feeding—this is true, due to the increase in calories being burned. You may have also heard that you can't lose *all* the baby weight while breast-feeding—this is also true. Some new mothers lose weight rapidly while breastfeeding, and some get stuck with the last few pounds, almost as a cushion for your newborn while you are breastfeeding. Everyone is different, and everyone's bodies react differently to breastfeeding. Don't be discouraged. The weight will come off as long as you eat right, exercise, and maintain a healthy lifestyle. If you decrease calories strictly, you will feel tired, especially if you are breastfeeding. You can begin exercising after 6 weeks, or when your health care provider tells you it is okay. In the meantime, you can do some light exercise, such as walking for 30 minutes a day, to build your muscle strength, get your blood circulation going, and to burn some extra calories.

After 6 to 8 weeks, when your body has somewhat recovered, you can consider some healthy weight-loss programs as long as your health care provider (and if you are breastfeeding, your pediatric health care provider) gives you the okay. If you diet too soon, your energy will be depleted, and you will feel tired and rundown, which can make your recovery take longer.

If you are planning on breastfeeding, you have to be a bit more careful when dieting is concerned, even after 6 weeks. There are some diet programs that have a breastfeeding plan. Weight Watchers, Medifast, and South Beach Phase 2 diet programs are all safe for breast-feeding moms. A lot of new moms are now using Shakeology shakes at http://www.shakeology.com/. Shakeology is a powdered shake full of nutritional supplements and super foods, such as protein, fiber, phyto-nutrients, vitamins, and minerals to fill you up and give you some energy throughout the day. Make sure that whatever plan you do choose is okay with your pediatric health care provider if you are breastfeeding. You will need enough calories and nutrients for energy and milk production. Whatever plan or program you choose, you should be receiving adequate amounts of nutrients from all of the food groups, and the weight loss should be slow and steady. Don't go on crash diets or drastically cut calories. You are still recovering, and will need a lot of energy throughout your baby's first year. Try not to restrict calories so much that you will cause a decrease in your milk supply.

There is no one-size-fits-all for diet and weight loss. Find a plan that is healthy and works for you, and stick to it. Remember that eating healthy and staying in shape is not a "diet" that will end when you have the results that you want— it is a way of life. Try to incorporate healthy eating into your lifestyle and it will evolve, as your newborn gets older, into a healthy lifestyle for your family. If you experienced cravings during pregnancy, and still crave sweets and fried foods, keep in mind that the more you eat healthy and avoid these foods, the less you will crave them. Satisfy your sweet cravings with some protein, a wedge of cheese, sliced turkey, or a handful of nuts. You can deviate from this way of eating and treat yourself once in a while, but make sure you go right back to it afterwards. You will notice that you don't feel right after bingeing on unhealthy foods once your body is used to eating right. As your baby grows, you will gain the desire and wisdom to continue to feed her healthy foods. Childhood obesity is increasing, and more and more children and adolescents are being diagnosed with diabetes and other childhood illnesses. Incorporating a healthy lifestyle for yourself while your baby is young will set a good healthy start for your family.

Drinking Enough Fluids

Thirst is a late sign of dehydration. You need to drink a certain amount of ounces of fluid for every pound of your body weight, roughly half of your body weight in ounces. For example if you weigh 150 pounds, you will need to drink at least 75 ounces of water per day. Breastfeeding will make you thirsty as a reminder to drink. It does not have to be strictly water. You can drink juices, which you can dilute with water (watch that you don't take in too much sugar), milk, broth, herbal teas, and soups. Purchase a water bottle that holds up to 64 ounces, and carry it with you throughout the day. You can add a squeeze of lemon juice, orange juice, sliced lemon, lime, or oranges to your water to add flavor. Foods, such as coffee, tea, alcohol and sodas are diuretics, which deplete water from your body. Observe your urine: if it is dark, concentrated, and amber colored, you are not getting enough water; if it is clear and light colored, you should be well hydrated.

Quick Healthy Meals and Snacks

- Hard-boiled eggs stored in a plastic container.

- Cut up vegetables, such as carrots, celery, peppers, beets, or cucumbers; eat plain, or dip in tahini or dressing.

- Cooked vegetables, such as asparagus, broccoli, cauliflower, or chilled steamed vegetables (good plain, or dipped in low-fat dressing, or in a salad).

- Canned tuna or salmon with cut up red onion and low-fat mayonnaise, salt, and pepper.

- Frozen, boneless chicken breasts in individual portions for quick grilling or baking with seasoning and olive oil.

- Nuts and seeds.

- Applesauce or yogurt, adding berries or granola to either.

- Smoothies: use milk (skim, coconut, soy, or almond), or fruit juice, 1-tablespoon nut butter, flax, or chia seeds, and a banana. You can add a protein shake with spirulina powder, whey, or egg powder for protein. Put all ingredients in a blender.

- A slice of whole-grain bread with nut butter, or slices of turkey.

- Grilled salmon with olive oil, salt and pepper, and brown rice.

- Soups: Buy a package or dry soup mix that contains most of the spices and ingredients you need for a good hearty soup. Just add onion, carrots, and broth, or, you can make your own and freeze.

- Use a slow cooker, or crock-pot. There are many recipes available in books or on the Internet. Throw in all the ingredients and it cooks itself. Use potatoes, vegetables, and a protein (meat cut up, or chicken), add some broth, and you have a whole meal a few hours later, with little effort. Perfect for the new mom!

► Pressure cookers are another way to get fast, easy meals that are delicious and full of protein. Dried beans are an excellent source of protein and can cook in 45 to 60 minutes in a pressure cooker. Pressure cookers are also great for making soup.

► Again, look on the Internet for recipes and ideas.

Vitamins and Minerals

Continue to take your prenatal vitamins, even if you are not breast-feeding. This will give you an extra balance of vitamins and minerals. Extra Vitamin D, especially in the winter months in the colder climates, is helpful for your mood, and helps to absorb calcium. You can take 2,000 IU (international units) per day, or more if your health care provider feels you will benefit from it.

Docosahexaenoic acid (DHA), a long-chain, omega-3 fatty acid, is good for your general health, but may also benefit your mood. You can get this from a supplement, fish, or foods fortified with DHA, such as eggs, soymilk, or orange juice. Be sure to read the package carefully to make sure it is DHA, and not general "omega-3s." Many prenatal vitamins contain DHA as it is a very important fat for you and for your newborn's developing brain. During your pregnancy, the placenta withdrew DHA from your body to supply the growing fetus. You need to replenish these stores or you can be compromised, emotionally and physically, during the postpartum period.

If you are anemic, you will need an iron supplement. Anemia can be due to your pregnancy itself causing a physiological anemia, or blood loss from the birth. Iron supplements, and foods containing iron, such as meats, organ meats, liver, spinach, egg yolks, and cream of wheat are all helpful to replenish your iron stores. Vitamin C also helps with iron absorption.

If you are a vegan and eat no animal products, you will need extra Vitamin B12. Check this with your health care provider. Make sure you consume enough protein. Legumes, nuts, tofu, whole grains, and rice, are all good foods for vegetarians. If you are vegan, and don't eat fish or eggs, you will also need iron supplements, as you need to be careful to avoid becoming anemic.

Constipation and Hemorrhoids

To help prevent and heal hemorrhoids, watch your diet and try to prevent constipation. Constipation can occur due to a number of reasons: not drinking enough fluids, taking narcotics for pain after birth, taking iron supplements, or having a sore perineum from an episiotomy that prevents you from straining or pushing. Exercise, eating healthy, non-constipating foods, drinking a lot of water and other fluids (such as prune juice), eating fiber-bran muffins, high-fiber cereals, fruits, vegetables, stool softeners, or osmotic laxatives, can all help reverse constipation. Try not to strain during a bowel movement, as this can aggravate or cause hemorrhoids to develop.

Ways to Alleviate Constipation

▶ Don't ignore the urge to have a bowel movement. The first one after your birth may be uncomfortable. The longer you wait, the harder the stool will be. Don't be afraid to push a little. You will not tear your stiches if you had an episiotomy. (You can try to support your perineum with a small towel or tissue paper while you push).

▶ Drink 6-8 glasses of water per day, or half your body weight in ounces.

▶ Drink straight prune juice, with the pulp.

▶ A warm liquid first thing in the morning, such as coffee, tea, or just plain warm water can help.

▶ Walk around the house to help stimulate your bowels.

▶ Dry fruit, such as raisins, dates, figs, apricots, or prunes are all good to eat and full of fiber.

- ▸ Take stool softeners, or whatever your health care provider prescribed.
- ▸ Relax. Do some pelvic-floor Kegels.
- ▸ Sit on the toilet, read a magazine, and give yourself time.

After-Baby Clothes

Although by now you will probably be sick and tired of your maternity clothes, and want to put them away for a very long time, you will still not be able to fit into your regular clothing for a little while. Once you return to your pre-baby weight, you can put away your maternity clothes for the next pregnancy, or give them away. Try and keep the ones that you purchased for special occasions, as you most likely can wear them again. For the time being, you can certainly look your best, and not spend a lot of money by purchasing some inexpensive, fitted, comfortable clothes. Two-piece outfits, such as tops, skirts, and pants, are more convenient than one-piece items, such as dresses, if you are breastfeeding, and for skin-to-skin if you are bottle-feeding.

There are many styles you can try that accentuate your good physical attributes and hide areas you don't want shown. Loose fitting tops will cover your belly: tunic sweaters, long cardigans, big sweaters and leggings; shirts that wrap around, or a wide belt can also hide areas you don't want revealed. Even though you don't plan on wearing these clothes for long, they are a good investment. Purchase a few items at a time, as your body will continue to change. Try some of the superstores, shop online, or buy a few things on the sale racks. During the first two weeks, it is okay to wear your pajamas and robe to remind yourself, and your visitors, that this is your time for healing and recuperation. After two weeks, do your hair, put on some makeup, and put on something clean and comfortable each day. By taking care of yourself, both inside and out, you will feel good and look good!

Healthy Snacks

- Raisins
- 100-Calorie packs
- Bananas
- Trail mix
- Peanuts
- Spirutein shakes
- Apples
- Protein bars
- Walnuts
- Rice cakes

- Pudding cups
- Applesauce
- Yogurt
- String cheese
- Grapes
- Cashews
- Lunch meat
- Granola bars
- Whole wheat breads

- Cheese cubes
- Peanut butter and crackers
- Cheerios
- Orange juice
- Baby carrots
- Apple juice
- Milk
- Hard-boiled eggs

*Postpartum Support International

Resources

Baby Center
http://www.babycenter.com/postpartum-health

USDA: Health and Nutrition Information for Pregnant and Breastfeeding Women
http://www.choosemyplate.gov/pregnancy-breastfeeding/breastfeeding-nurtitional-needs.html

Foodpyramid.com
http://www.foodpyramid.com/myplate/for-moms/

NHS Choices: *Your health, your choices*
http://www.nhs.uk/conditions/pregnancy-and-baby/pages/keeping-fit-and-healthy.aspx#close

WomensHealth.Gov: Office on women's health, U.S. department of health and human services
http://www.womenshealth.gov/pregnancy/childbirth-beyond/recovering-from-birth.html

Chapter 7
Post-Baby Love and Sex

"What is the safest time to resume having sex?"
"When will I feel like having sex again?"

Love and Sex after Birth

As a new mother, with a brand-new baby to care for 24/7, sex is probably the last thing on your mind (Although your partner may have a different idea). You will be facing many new challenges concerning sex and intimacy after giving birth. You may be dealing with soreness, stitches, sleep deprivation, time constraints, and overwhelming fatigue. You may have concerns regarding hemorrhoids, your episiotomy or cesarean incision, or simply be fearful of your first time having sex after birth. You may be concerned about your decreased interest or desire, as well as whether or not you will experience pain, and, if so, for how long. Nonetheless, sexuality is a very important component of your physical and psychological well-being for both you and your partner.

When Can We Start?

Depending on how you are feeling, how much lochia bleeding you are experiencing, and instructions from your health care provider, the time you need to wait to resume sexual activity can vary. For the first 3 to 6 weeks, you are expelling products of conception in your lochia and, if you had an episiotomy, you are still healing on the outside. You may wish to wait until your 6-week postpartum checkup. Typically, it is safe to resume sex when you and your partner feel it is the right time. However, it is imperative you at least wait until your bleeding has ceased. If you are still bleeding, you are not yet completely healed on the inside.

You also need to consider whether your body has healed on the outside. If you had an episiotomy, a perineal tear, or a cesarean section, and you wait until your incision has healed, sex will be easier for you. An episiotomy can take 6 to 8 weeks—or longer—to heal. For the first few months, intercourse may still be a little bit uncomfortable. Even after your stitches have healed, you may be a little sore at first. As time goes on, the scar tissue will stretch itself out, and you should not experience any more discomfort during sex. It takes time for your perineum to stretch and become more pliable. A cesarean section scar will take anywhere from 6 to 8 weeks to heal, depending on the type of incision, but you may still experience some discomfort for a few months after this initial healing phase. Finding the right position where you do not feel pressure on your stitches or scars can help make sex more enjoyable for you and your partner.

Many postpartum couples will have resumed lovemaking by 3 months postpartum, but this number varies, and every couple is different. It is important for you to talk to your partner about your feelings regarding either resuming sexual activity, or your desire to wait. There are alternative ways of maintaining intimacy that you can try during this time until you are ready for intercourse. Try to get some rest, drink plenty of fluids, and eat well so you can have the energy and strength to resume your sexual relationship.

I Have No Desire For Sex. Is This Normal?

Your passion for lovemaking may be lower than usual after giving birth. This is quite common, as your body and emotions have been through a tremendous change. You need time to heal, from the inside and the outside, physically and psychologically. You may be ready to resume having sex after 3 to 6 weeks, or you may not be ready for a few months. Aside from the physical reasons for having a low libido, there are also emotional reasons for not being very interested in sex. Having your newborn hanging on your breasts all day can certainly decrease your desire to have someone else touch or fondle them. You are now preoccupied with your newborn, and may be afraid he will wake up during sex, or that you won't hear crying or fussing. You may have spit up all over your clothes and you may not have had the time to shower, let alone make yourself feel attractive. If you experienced a difficult birth, or any type of trauma during childbirth, you might need time to heal emotionally and feel comfortable with your body again before you can rediscover your sexual self.

Reasons for a Low Sex Drive

A decline in sexual interest after the birth of your newborn is perfectly normal and can be due to a number of factors.

- Fatigue, exhaustion
- Feeling overwhelmed
- Hearing your baby crying may spoil the mood
- Fear that you won't hear the baby
- Difficulty adjusting to your new parenting role
- Hormonal changes, such as a sudden drop in estrogen and progesterone
- Vaginal dryness due to declining estrogen levels
- Physical discomfort in your vulva, vagina, perineum, breasts, or abdomen
- Fear of milk leakage from breasts
- Feeling self-conscious about your body image and the changes in your body
- Sleep deprivation may reduce desire or response to stimulation
- Adjustment to new motherhood

Rediscovering your Sexual Desire

Sex after the birth of your newborn takes on a completely new dimension now that you both are parents. You and your partner, as a couple, have a product of your love—your new baby. You will need to be creative during this time as you become closer than ever before, sharing in one of the greatest miracles of life. You have reproduced together, and you will work to make it through this challenging time while you reenergize your passion for each other.

The first few times you have sex, you might experience vaginal dryness, tightness or looseness, bleeding or irritation, and discomfort or pain in the perineal area from your stitches. You may have a decrease in vaginal lubrication, especially if you are breastfeeding. This is due to the decline in estrogen after birth. Your vaginal tissue is also a little thinner than before, which can also lead to vaginal discomfort during sex. These discomforts should resolve over time as the vagina and perineum relaxes and stretches. There are several over-the-counter vaginal lubricants you can try to ease the pain or discomfort. However, if pain persists, see your health care provider. If your vagina feels loose, you can try some Kegel exercises, and, over time, your vagina will regain its muscle tone.

If you are breastfeeding, milk can spurt from your nipples due to the release of oxytocin during sex or orgasm. You may not care, or find this amusing or pleasurable, or you may be embarrassed by this and choose to wear a bra during lovemaking. If you feed your baby beforehand, it will reduce the chances of milk release. Initially, you may have more discomfort than pleasure, but give yourself time and be patient. It will get better, and your sex life will get back to what it used to be.

You can express your sexuality in many ways besides through sexual intercourse. You can satisfy each other with lovemaking that does not involve penetration. It is possible to achieve sexual fulfillment even during the times when intercourse is not an option or is not advised. It may have been a while since you have been able to have sexual intercourse. You may have had preterm labor contractions, your water may have broken, or you might have been very uncomfortable during your pregnancy. As a couple, you can find pleasure from other activities that do not involve intercourse.

Be patient and communicate with each other. Reassure yourselves that you that you are a team, and you are both working together to care for your newborn and raise your new family. Explore other ways to maintain intimacy. Sex is also about closeness, communication, and pleasuring one another. You and your partner can maintain intimacy through kissing, touching, cuddling, hugging, massaging each other, or simply holding hands. For sexual pleasure, you can try stroking or oral sex.

When You Are Ready

- No sex until all bleeding has ceased (lochia is a sign that you are not done healing).

- For discomfort or pain in the vagina due to dryness, or perineum due to episiotomy, use vaginal lubricant, and experiment with positions that put less pressure on stitches or soreness and let you control penetration.

- For breast tenderness, be gentle. You can wear a bra for support and to prevent leakage during sex if breastfeeding (feed baby beforehand to decrease chance of leakage).

- To avoid fatigue, try to get some rest beforehand and plan ahead.

- Use contraception. Your body needs to heal and recover. Another pregnancy too soon can be taxing on your body.

- Warm up with foreplay and give yourself time.

- Have a glass of wine or herbal tea to relax beforehand.

- Give each other a massage with scented oils, or light some scented candles to relax and get yourself in the mood.

- Take it slow, and find a time when you do not feel rushed.

- Kegel exercises beforehand and during can help bring blood flow to your perineum for healing and make the muscles flexible.

Warning Signs

- Painful intercourse
- Foul-smelling vaginal discharge

- Bleeding after 4 to 6 weeks, or a sudden increase in bleeding
- Fever over 100.4° F
- Pain or burning when urinating

Making it Work

The first 6 weeks postpartum can put your relationship with your partner to the test. This can be a tough time in your lives together as a couple. It can make you closer, or pull you apart. The demands and pressures of caring for a newborn can cause stress between the two of you even though you love each other very much and want to be there for each other. Parenthood is a huge adjustment as you are learning your place and role as parents.

The birth of your newborn, especially if it is your first, is the biggest transition you and your partner will ever face as a couple. It is the biggest joy, but can also come with mixed emotions. Your life is no longer your own. You are completely responsible for another human being, and that responsibility doesn't end when your shift is up. Although you may have talked about becoming parents for 9 months—or even longer—once your newborn is in your arms, you may have completely different views and feelings than you did before. I have seen new mothers who were completely career driven, with plans to return to work as soon as they could, change their minds when their newborn arrived and quit their jobs to be stay-at-home moms. I have also seen the complete opposite: women who were planning to be stay-at-home moms deciding it was not for them, return to work.

Regarding work, childcare, and raising your baby, it is important to be on the same page with your partner. Don't forget who you are as a couple and as sexual partners. You may have to work at this a little bit harder now. Taking time out for yourselves for romance and alone time is crucial for your marriage. There will be times over the next weeks, months, and even years where you will forget that you were once a romantic couple. Putting in effort early is a way to maintain romance and sexuality so that you don't lose sight of it later on. Remind yourselves that you are a couple, and you need this time alone. You both still need affection, love, and intimacy from each other.

Share your thoughts and feelings about your new lives and your transition to parenthood. It might sound silly, but you may well need to schedule your times together. The two of you can take a walk alone in the evening if you have a babysitter, or take your newborn with you in a stroller. You can sit down and have a cup of tea together before you go to bed, once your newborn has gone to sleep. If your newborn is fussy and likes the motion of the car, go for a drive. You can get ice cream, or a latte, and sit in the car while he is sleeping. Talk about the changes in your lives and ask your partner if he or she is feeling a lack of attention. Think of small ideas to keep your romance alive. You could have a date night at home with a candlelit dinner, or you can hire a babysitter once or twice a month, and go out. Take a bath together or give each other a massage. Enlist grandparents, neighbors, nieces or nephews, or other friends or family to help out. More important than having sex is that you communicate and be present for each other. Staying emotionally connected is just as important, if not more, than being physically connected. Work on your relationship, and your love for each other will continue to grow and flourish.

Post-Baby Birth Control

There are many myths regarding fertility after birth. The last thing that you, as a new mother, want is to become pregnant again during the first 6 weeks postpartum. But that can certainly happen. Breastfeeding can postpone pregnancy, but it is a myth that you cannot conceive while breastfeeding. Breastfeeding regularly can inhibit ovulation and fertility, and you will have a delay in menstruation due to the increase in prolactin. This may decrease your chance of conceiving, however, as time goes on, if you have fewer feedings and limited nighttime breastfeeding, it will not be a reliable means of contraception.

Keep in mind that you will ovulate before you menstruate and may not know that you are ovulating. You can become pregnant during that time before your period returns. Women have become pregnant while breastfeeding, therefore you may wish to use a backup method of birth control. Formula-feeding mothers will usually begin menstruating by 3 months postpartum. Breastfeeding mothers may begin menstruation at this time as well, or it may take up to a year for menstruation to return.

What type of birth control should I consider?
If I am breastfeeding, what are my options?

Choices for Contraception

There are a large variety of contraceptive choices for you as a new mother. However, the choices are fewer if you are breastfeeding. There are hormonal, non-hormonal, barrier, and permanent methods of birth control. Non-hormonal, or very-low-hormone contraceptives are recommended if you are breastfeeding. Non-hormonal contraceptive options include condoms, diaphragms, cervical caps, spermicides, some intrauterine devices (IUDs), and natural family planning. Permanent, non-hormonal methods would include tubal ligation for yourself or a vasectomy for your partner.

There are two types of hormonal contraception: those with estrogen and progesterone, and those with progesterone only. Some of these hormones pass into breast milk, so it is safest to use progesterone-only options while breastfeeding. Either contraceptive method can decrease your milk supply, so it is best if you start progesterone-only birth control after you've established a good milk supply and your newborn is gaining weight. Avoid contraceptives with estrogen, as these can cause your milk supply to drop.

The progesterone-only pill is also called the mini pill. You can also receive progesterone as an injection, IUD, or implant. Depo-Provera is an injectable form of progesterone that lasts for three months. You can also use Norplant, which is a progesterone implant in your arm, which lasts five years. There is also a progesterone IUD called Mirena.

It may be a good idea to wait at least 2 to 3 weeks postpartum, until your milk supply is established, before taking the mini pill, injectable, or implantable progesterone-based method of contraception. Before using one of the more permanent progesterone methods, you can try the mini pill to see if the progesterone will affect your milk supply. Combined estrogen and progesterone methods come in a pill, a patch that you apply every week for three weeks per month, a ring inserted into the vagina each month that you leave in for three weeks, or as a monthly injection. Avoid birth control options with estrogen if you are breastfeeding.

If you have had unprotected sex and fear you may have conceived, you can use the morning after pill, also known as emergency contraception, or Plan-B. Although it may make you slightly nauseated, and should not be used frequently, it is considered to be safe if you are breastfeeding. You can refer to the chart below for more information regarding different options for birth control. Speak to your health care provider about making the right choice that is best for you, your partner, and your baby (McDonald & Brown, 2013).

Contraception Options for the Postpartum Mom

(Sober & Schreiber, 2014; Birth control methods fact sheet. http://www.womenshealth. gov/publications/our-publications/fact-sheet/birth-control-methods.html, 2012; http://www.infantrisk.com/content/safe-use-birth-control-while-breastfeeding, 2015)

Method	Effectiveness Rate-Perfect use; typical use	Recommended during breastfeeding	Advantages	Disadvantages	Hormones
Natural Family Planning (Methods that do not involve any chemicals or insertion of foreign objects)					
Lactation Amenorrhea Method (LAM)	95%-99% up to six months; 5% after six months	Yes	Completely Natural	Requires round the clock breast-feeding with no supplements (does not include expressing and pumping). Menses has not returned.	No
Coitus Interruptus (withdrawal)	78%	Yes	Natural, no cost	Sperm may be present prior to ejaculation; interrupts spontaneity	No
Fertility Aware-ness Methods: Basal Body Temperature Method (BBT) Cervical Mucus Method (Billings method) Ovulation method (kits), Calendar Method	76%	Yes	Natural, no cost	Need motivation, preparation and planning; can interrupt spontaneity	No

Method	Effectiveness Rate-Perfect use; typical use	Recommended during breastfeeding	Advantages	Disadvantages	Hormones
		Barrier methods			
Male condom	84%	Yes	No effect on breast milk or baby; can use lubricated condoms to help with vaginal dryness; easy to use and purchase	May interrupt spontaneity	No
Female Condom	79%	Yes	Can be inserted 8 hours prior to sex; no effect on breast milk or baby	Insertion can be challenging	No
Spermicide (alone)	74%	Yes	No effect on breast milk or baby	Must be inserted 5-10 minutes before sex; can develop sensitivity; can have a discharge afterwards	No
Diaphragm with spermicide	88%	Yes	Easy to insert; no effect on breast milk or baby	Must be refitted after birth or weight loss; needs to be left in place six hours after sex, can cause irritation, discharge; prescription needed; watch for Toxic Shock Syndrome (TSS)	No

Method	Effectiveness Rate-Perfect use; typical use	Recommended during breastfeeding	Advantages	Disadvantages	Hormones
Cervical cap with spermicide	60%-80%	Yes	Can leave in place for a few days; less spermicide than with diaphragm; no effect on spontaneity	Difficult insertion or removal; can cause irritation to cervix; can cause allergic reaction; watch for TSS	No
Intrauterine Device (IUD) (non-hormonal)	99.2%	Yes	Can be inserted by health care provider early after delivery; no interruption or reminder needed	Possible increase in bleeding and cramping during menses	No
Hormonal methods: Progesterone Only					
IUD with hormones	99,9%	With Caution; must wait until 6 weeks after delivery	Progesterone only; Can be inserted by health care provider early after delivery; no interruption or reminder needed	Although less than without hormones, possible increase in bleeding and cramping during menses	Yes
Mini-Pill (progestin only oral contraception)	92%	With Caution; Must wait until 6 weeks after delivery	No effect on baby; minimal side effects	Can decrease milk supply; must be taken at exactly same time each day	Yes
Depo Provera	99.7%	With Caution; hormones can be transmitted to baby; can start 6 weeks after birth	Lasts 3 months; no interruption in spontaneity	Need injection every 3 months; can delay future fertility up to 9 months; no period while using this method; weight gain	Yes

Method	Effectiveness Rate-Perfect use; typical use	Recommended during breastfeeding	Advantages	Disadvantages	Hormones
Intradermal Implant	99.9%	With caution	Lasts up to 3 years	Initial cost; insertion and removal can be uncomfort-able; can see implants on arm	Yes
Hormonal methods: Estrogen and Progesterone					
Contraceptive Skin Patch	92%	Not recom-mended: may affect milk supply and baby	Easy to use, worn for 3 weeks each month; does not interrupt spontaneity	Contains estrogen and progesterone; higher risk of blood clots than with birth control pills; can cause skin irritation	Yes
Vaginal Ring (NuvaRing)	92%	Not recom-mended: May affect milk supply and baby	Easy to use and insert; worn for 3 weeks; does not interrupt spontaneity	Contains estrogen and progesterone; risk of blood clots; need to remember to insert	Yes
Oral Contracep-tives	97%	Not recom-mended: May affect milk supply and baby	Does not interrupt spontaneity	Contains estrogen and progesterone; risk of blood clots; risk of thrombophle-bitis	Yes
Surgical Methods					
Tubal Ligation	99.5%	Yes	Permanent; very reliable; Does not interrupt spontaneity	Most likely irreversible; surgical procedure	No
Vasectomy	99.5%	Yes	Permanent; very reliable; Does not interrupt spontaneity	Most likely irreversible; surgical procedure	No

Method	Effectiveness Rate-Perfect use; typical use	Recommended during breastfeeding	Advantages	Disadvantages	Hormones
Emergency Contraception					
Morning-after pill or Plan B	89%	Probably will not affect breast milk; High dose of birth control may affect baby (pump and dump for 8 hours to limit baby's exposure to the hormones;	Easy to obtain, over the counter	Must be taken within 72 hours of unprotected sex; Nausea, vomiting	Yes, high doses

Resources

Office of Women's Health (2011). *Birth control methods fact sheet.*
Retrieved from http://www.womenshealth.gov/publications/our-publications/fact-sheet/birth-control-methods.html

InfantRisk.com. (2011). *Safe use of birth control while breastfeeding.*
Retrieved from http://www.infantrisk.com/content/safe-use-of-birth-control-while-breastfeeding.

CDC Center for disease control and prevention.
http://www.cdc.gov/reproductivehealth/UnintendedPregnancy/Contraception.htm

Let's talk about sex: After the baby
http://www.babycenter.com/0_lets-talk-about-sex-after-the-baby_11802.bc

Your sex life after baby
http://www.webmd.com/parenting/baby/features/your-sex-life-after-baby

Planned Parenthood
http://www.plannedparenthood.org/health-info/birth-control

Chapter 8
Postpartum Dad

As a new father, you may also find that becoming a parent for the first time can be overwhelming. You may find yourself wondering what exactly your role is. Nowadays, fathers are much more involved than they used to be. Dads spend more time with their children, and they are involved with their children's sports and other activities. Caring for your newborn will help you feel closer to your child. The relationship you formulate now will set the stage for when your child is older. There is, however, a learning curve, and bonding with your child does take time. Reading up on newborn care, and talking to other new fathers, including your own can make you feel more prepared (Sears, Sears, Sears, & Sears, 2013).

Many new fathers have never had the opportunity to see or hold a newborn baby. You may only have experience with older babies, who are larger and cuter, and can respond to people by smiling or cooing, such as those seen in movies or television commercials. Even "newborn babies" in movies, are usually much older babies. A brand-new baby will look very different, and may appear smaller and more fragile than you expect, and you may feel a little disappointed at first. She doesn't resemble you or your partner, may have a "cone head" from being pushed out, has an umbilical cord stump with a clamp, may have black hair or a cheesy substance all over her body, and is a ruddy color, with puffy eyes, and wrinkly skin.

Don't feel let down by your newborn's appearance, as she will grow and change quickly. One day, you may think she resembles you, while the next day you may think she looks more like your partner or another relative. Every day, you will see changes in your newborn, and the features you and your partner have will begin to emerge.

Adjusting to a newborn can be challenging for both of you. You need to adjust to many new responsibilities, and may feel overwhelmed—especially during the first 6 weeks. Not only will you be caring for your newborn, but you may also be caring for your partner, especially if she has had a cesarean birth. Your routine, sleep, and daily activities will all be disrupted. A typical day with a newborn includes:

- Feeding 8 to 12 times a day
- Burping in between and after feedings
- Changing diapers 8 to 12 times per day
- A bath or sponge bath at least once per day
- Soothing when fussy
- Preparing and sterilizing bottles of formula if your partner is bottle-feeding
- Helping your partner pump and store milk for future use, if breastfeeding

Your newborn will create her own schedule. For the first 6 weeks, it may seem as if all she does is eat, sleep, wet, poop, cry, and fuss. Both you and your partner need sleep and rest. Take turns either getting up with her or napping to get some extra sleep. Ask family and friends to help with meals, cleaning, laundry, and watching your newborn so you both can rest.

My Partner Is Breastfeeding? What Is My Role?

There may be times when you may feel like a third wheel, especially if your partner is breastfeeding. You are certainly not an outsider—you nurtured your partner and unborn baby during pregnancy, and you will continue to do so in the days and weeks to come. If she is breastfeeding, she still needs your help and support (Hunter & Cattelona, 2014). You were a vital part of the birthing process, and are now a vital part of the postpartum experience. Get involved and get your hands dirty—there is plenty that you can do. Breastfeeding is often not easy for the new mother, and she will need plenty of support and encouragement. You, as the baby's other parent, are the best person for this job.

Supporting the Breastfeeding Dyad

- ▸ Provide mom with some comfort. If you see she is having a difficult time with positioning, offer her a pillow for under her arm or behind her back for extra support.

- ▸ Bring her a glass or bottle of water, as she needs the fluids, and will be thirsty while she is breastfeeding.

- ▸ Encourage her, especially if she has had a difficult birth, and is having a difficult time.

- ▸ Encourage relaxation. You can lower her stress level by taking care of things around the house while she is breastfeeding.

- ▸ Bring her a snack if she has not had the chance to eat.

- ▸ Bring your newborn to and from your partner for feedings so she doesn't have to get up, especially if she is uncomfortable after childbirth.

- ▸ Once your partner's milk supply is established (after about 2 to 3 weeks), you can even feed your newborn pumped breast milk in a bottle to allow the breastfeeding mother a good stretch of sleep.

- ▸ Change diapers.

- ▸ Do the burping in between and after feedings.

- ▸ Wear your newborn in a sling or carrier so that your partner can get some rest.

- ▸ Soothe your fussy newborn by rocking, walking, reading, or singing to her, or holding her skin to skin.

- ▸ Bathe your baby.

These are all good ways to not only support your partner, but to bond with your newborn. Spending time with mother and baby together, as well as separately, is a good way to form a family bond. If you are bottle-feeding your newborn, you can certainly share in all aspects of feeding.

Dad and Baby Bonding

You may not feel an instant connection with your newborn, and that is completely normal. The same is true for the new mother. Bonding with your newborn does not always happen right away, especially during the first 6 weeks. You may feel as if your newborn does not respond to you. However, your newborn is actually aware of your scent, touch, and voice. You will feel much closer to your newborn once she starts to recognize you, smile at you, gets excited when she sees you, or put her arms out for you to hold her.

Men bond with their babies differently than women do, and babies know the difference. You can be proactive by reading, learning, and practicing. Accompanying your partner and newborn to the pediatric health care provider will allow you to learn more about your newborn and her development. Try and carve out some time for yourself as well. Between work, baby, and partner, you need some alone time too.

Responding to your newborn's cries during the day and night will help make you feel connected and a vital part of your newborn's life, as your partner is not the only one who can soothe her (Kotila & Kamp Dush, 2012). Learning some baby-care basics will help you to feel closer and more involved with your newborn's care. Learn how to swaddle, and hold your baby often; they are not as fragile as you think.

Stay-at-Home-Dad (SAHD)

More and more fathers are becoming primary caregivers for a variety of reasons (Durante, Griskevicius, Simpson, Cantú, & Tybur, 2012). It's not a bad choice for you—a relaxed dress code, flexible work schedule, and spending time outdoors. You may be working from home and caring for your baby at the same time, or you may be in between jobs, allowing your partner the opportunity to develop her career without worrying about childcare. Being a SAHD is a wonderful opportunity to bond with your baby while giving yourself time to do something different. Connecting with other SAHDs, or even stay-at-home mothers, will offer you and your baby some socialization, and help make you feel less isolated. Try to break up the day by going on outings, joining a class as your baby gets older, and planning for activities. Most of all, cherish this time with your baby and feel lucky that you have this wonderful opportunity to take part in her day-to-day care and watch her grow.

Basic Baby Care Techniques

Diapering

Your newborn can have 6 to 8 wet diapers, and 3 to 4 bowel movements per day. If breastfeeding, this number can be even higher.

- ▸ Make sure you have all the supplies you need ready and on hand.

- ▸ Put the baby on a changing table, on her back. Never turn away when changing your baby, and always have one hand above your baby in case they move or roll over.

- ▸ Unfasten the dirty diaper tabs. To prevent them from sticking to your baby, fold them over. Hold the baby's two ankles together. Use the front half of the diaper to wipe off any stool from his or her bottom. Fold the dirty diaper in half underneath your baby, with the clean side up.

- ▸ Lift your newborn up slightly, and with the other hand, use a baby wipe, cleaning from front to back and then patting dry with a cloth diaper or washcloth.

- ▸ Slide a clean diaper (tabs in the back) under baby's bottom, and apply powder or diaper rash cream. For boys, clean under scrotum, as there may be more stool there.

- ▸ Pull the front half of the diaper up to your baby's belly, folding over so the cord stump is exposed.

- ▸ Fasten and secure the diaper at both sides with the tabs, not too tightly, making sure there are no open spaces near the legs.

- ▸ If using cloth diapers, the procedure is the same, using a diaper cover with Velcro.

There are many advantages to using cloth diapers. You can wash the diapers yourself or use a diaper service. There is a lower risk of diaper rash, you can save money, there is no exposure to chemicals found in disposable diapers, they are better for the environment and create less trash, you will not need to make midnight runs to the store because you ran out of diapers, and they have easy to use liner pants that fasten with Velcro. You should not use old-fashioned diaper pins, as they can become unfastened and injure your baby.

Swaddling your Newborn

What does swaddle mean?
What is the advantage to swaddling?

Swaddling a newborn is the art of snuggly wrapping your newborn in a blanket for warmth and security, mimicking being in the womb. Because your newborn will feel secure, it helps to calm her. You can swaddle your newborn for the first 6 to 8 weeks. After this time, most infants will become acclimated to life outside of the womb and will not need the security of the swaddle. In addition, she will need to be free to move around at night and stretch. The benefits to swaddling your newborn are that she will sleep better and longer, cry and fuss less, have a diminished startle reflex, and won't scratch herself with her nails.

How to Swaddle

- ▸ Spread out a thin receiving blanket in a diamond shape, folding one corner down.
- ▸ Lay your baby face up, placing the head at the edge of the folded corner, arms at their sides.
- ▸ Fold the top right across baby's body with their arm down, tucking the blanket under her left side.
- ▸ Fold the bottom point of the blanket up, leaving room for the feet to move freely, tucking the corner under the left armpit.
- ▸ Pick up the left side of the blanket and bring across baby's body, tucking the blanket on the right side.

▸ Never place your newborn on her stomach. Instead, place on her back or side.

The Newborn Bath

Some people feel that it is not necessary to bathe a baby every day. Others feel that because their babies get so dirty from spit up and soiled diapers that they wish to bathe them daily. It is a personal choice, and there is no harm in bathing once a day, or three times a week.

▸ Use a small plastic baby tub or a clean sink. The room should be nice and warm.

▸ Gather all your supplies, including a soft blanket, a hooded towel, a clean diaper, and pajamas.

▸ You will only need 2 to 3 inches of warm water (about 90 degrees F, 32 Celsius; test on your wrist to make sure it is not too hot). To keep baby warm, pour warm water over her body throughout the bath.

▸ Undress baby and slip into the tub feet first, using one hand to support the back and neck, and the other hand to bathe.

▸ Start with only warm water on a washcloth to wipe eyes, from the corners to the outside, and then the face. Using mild baby soap, wash with your hand or a washcloth from top to bottom, cleaning the diaper area last.

▸ Rinse baby thoroughly with warm water.

▸ You can wash baby's hair while in the bath, or wrap baby in a towel to dry and gently wash hair while holding over the sink or bath, then gently dry hair with a cloth or towel.

▸ Apply mild baby lotion and dress in warm pajamas.

Some newborns like the bath, and others don't. Your newborn may cry the entire time, but will get used to her bath over time.

Burping

- Put your newborn's head on your shoulder, with your arm under her bottom, or ...

- Lean her body forward to support the chest and chin with one hand and rub her back with the other, or ...

- Sit baby on your lap or lay across your lap face down, supporting chest and head.

- Use opposite arm to rub baby's back.

Post-Baby Relationship

It takes time, practice, and work to maintain your strong connection as a couple. Be considerate of each other, and don't forget to communicate. Work together as parents, and as a team. Parenting duties are hard work, but will also bring you a lot of joy. You may choose to do certain things differently than your partner does. Find ways to accept each other's routine as long as neither routine is unsafe. You will not always agree on everything. Try to be flexible and support each other, even if your way of doing things is different. Compliment each other and try and see each other's point of view. Work together to maintain your relationship and talk about your feelings.

During the first 6 weeks of being a new dad, try to be available as much as possible. Hopefully, you are able to take off a week or two from work, or, if you can afford it, can take an unpaid leave. If you can't do either, try to be home early, don't plan business trips during this time, or late nights at the office, if at all possible. Try not to make plans for the first few weeks when your partner is recovering. Pitch in with household tasks and caring for your baby when you are home. You may not get to relax in the evening until all the tasks are done and your baby has gone to sleep. You may begin to wonder what you did with your time before your baby was born. You may feel as if your new life is unrecognizable, and that you're completely surrounded by new responsibilities. Although this lifestyle change can be overwhelming in the beginning, it is temporary. You will slowly begin to enjoy the things that you did before, but for now, let your partner and baby know that you are there for them.

Be open to hiring a postpartum doula, especially if your family is not nearby, or you have no relatives that can come and help you during this time. A postpartum doula can help you, the dad, as well. She can teach you how to support the new mother, and help with laundry, dishes, and basic baby care, or give you a break so you can run out to the store. Just as your partner has to learn how to be a mom, you have to learn how to be a dad. It takes time, just like any new skill you may have mastered. You will make mistakes and you will learn from them.

Her Postpartum Emotions

Please read Chapter 9 on postpartum or perinatal mood disorders (PPMD), and be aware of the possible signs and symptoms of PPMD. If you feel your partner is exhibiting any of the signs, such as baby blues that do not go away after 2 weeks, depression and/or anxiety, not sleeping or sleeping too much, not eating, extreme worry or not showing interest in the newborn, or fear of harming herself or her newborn, please take her to get help. You can ask your obstetrician, doula, or lactation consultant for a recommendation. Find a therapist who specializes in PPMD, or look on the web. Postpartum Support International (PSI) has coordinators who can put you on the right path for a specialist in your area, along with chat rooms, and online support for mothers and fathers. Even if she does not want to go, make an appointment and bring her. Ways to help her recover quickly and help prevent PPMD are:

- ▸ Help with household and newborn care.
- ▸ Allow her to take breaks from the baby.
- ▸ Make sure she has adequate fluids.
- ▸ Ensure she gets three full balanced meals a day.
- ▸ Have her avoid caffeine and too much sugar.
- ▸ Encourage her to get out of the house at least once a day.
- ▸ Make sure she has social support.

Resources

Focus on the Family
www.focusonthefamily.com/parenting

National Center for Fathering
www.fathers.com

National Fatherhood Initiative
www.fatherhood.org

PostpartumDads: Helping Families Overcome Postpartum Depression (PPD)
http://www.postpartumdads.org/

Chapter 9
Post-Baby Mood Disorders

"I am just not feeling like myself.
Could I have postpartum depression?"

"What exactly is postpartum depression?"

"I love my baby— how can
I be feeling depressed?"

"How can I cope with this?"

The first 6 weeks after giving birth are the most difficult and demanding weeks that you will ever experience. This time period is draining, both physically and mentally. The amount of stress that you, as a laboring woman have just been through, is exhausting, not to mention the hormonal changes that your body has gone through as a result. During pregnancy, hormonal levels of estrogen and progesterone increase drastically. These are considered to be the main hormones of pregnancy, and they typically, but not always, have a positive effect on a pregnant woman's mood. These hormones produce the notorious "glow" of pregnancy, helping the fetus to develop properly. Some women feel good during this time. However, others can develop significant symptoms of depression and anxiety during pregnancy. This often depends a lot on their prior personal or family history of depression and anxiety and their risk factors. (Buttner, O'Hara, & Watson, 2012). Immediately after delivery, these hormones decrease rapidly. These hormones will usually take a few weeks to regulate, a little longer if you are breastfeeding. The new hormones that take over during this time are oxytocin and prolactin.

I cry more than my baby does.

As a new mother, you may find yourself crying over a sensitive commercial, bursting into tears when your partner asks you a simple question, or crying for no reason at all. You are worrying about your baby, unable to sleep even though exhausted, and you are overly concerned about being a good mother. These are just some of the emotional symptoms that many new mothers experience.

> *I'm having a hard time concentrating. I can't read more than a few words of a book, newspaper, or magazine.*

These symptoms can be caused by exhaustion or sleep deprivation, which can also leave you feeling anxious about caring for your baby.

> *What does the baby want?*
> *Why is he still crying after being fed and changed?*
> *Why can't I get him to sleep?*

You may be struggling with not knowing what your baby needs or wants, not knowing why he is crying or fussing. You may be trying to learn how to get your baby to sleep. In the few hours that your baby sleeps during the day, you may try to rush around getting chores done because you don't know how long the sleep will last.

In the evening, not knowing how many hours the baby will sleep at night may cause you some anxiety, so that you can't fall asleep when the baby is sleeping. If you were not the type of person who could fall asleep at will, you may have trouble falling asleep as soon as the baby does, or may have trouble falling back to sleep after a feeding. Some new mothers are so stressed about lack of sleep that they can't fall asleep at all, and become increasingly anxious about sleep in general. This can sometimes lead to a vicious cycle of insomnia and sleep deprivation.

After birthing a baby, even if the birth was relatively easy, you may experience physical discomfort along with some level of emotional turmoil. You are probably sleep deprived and may be experiencing pain or discomfort from the episiotomy stitches, perineal tears, or just the physical trauma of birth. You may be having afterbirth pains and breast soreness, even if breastfeeding is going well.

If breastfeeding is challenging for you and your baby, you may begin to feel even more overwhelmed. Your body is recovering from a decline in vitamins and minerals, specifically iron, due to the afterbirth bleeding, lochia discharge, and what's known as physiological anemia during pregnancy. This condition is caused by a dilution of red blood cells during pregnancy, which lowers the hemoglobin and hematocrit count, giving you temporary anemia. This often resolves after birth, but together with excess loss of blood, can make you feel fatigued and drained. Your body needs at least 6 to 8 weeks to recover from these physiological changes, blood and fluid losses, and the physical muscular strain of delivery.

All of these circumstances, plus a combination of hormonal fluctuations, electrolyte imbalance, sleep deprivation, exhaustion, psychological adjustment, social pressure, social comparison, and the expectation that everything needs to be perfect, can all contribute to a "perfect storm," setting off Postpartum/Perinatal Mood Disorders (PPMD) (Bennett & Indman, 2015; Kleiman & Wenzel, 2014).

What are Postpartum and Perinatal Mood Disorders (PPMD)?

PPMD are the most common complication of childbirth today. It is a biochemical illness, affecting many aspects of your psychological and physical well-being. They make you question your ability to care for yourself and your newborn. PPMD may also cause you to question your own sanity and can be extremely frightening for any new mother.

Approximately 15 to 25 percent of postpartum women will experience some form of PPMD. This number does not include those that suffer in silence because they fear coming forward, and therefore do not get the help they need. It does not include those new mothers who simply do not know or understand why they are feeling this way, and just muddle through it. Perinatal depression and anxiety are the most undertreated illnesses, and one of the most underreported mental illnesses, in our society. PPMD not only affects the new mother, but the baby, her partner, and the entire family. With proper diagnosis and treatment, you will get better with a little bit of time. Typically, treatment includes psychotherapy, medication, non-pharmacological supplements, and alternative treatments, or a combination of methods (Puryear, 2007; Scharff, 2004; Zauderer & Davis, 2012).

PPD/PPMD is an umbrella term that describes a cluster of symptoms and can be broken down further into several categories:

- ▸ Postpartum depression
- ▸ Postpartum anxiety, including panic disorders, and obsessive compulsive disorders
- ▸ Postpartum post-traumatic stress disorder.
- ▸ Bipolar Disorder and Postpartum psychosis.

What are "Baby Blues?"

Postpartum blues or baby blues affect many new mothers and are often considered a normal adjustment to new motherhood, although there can be some overlap with PPMD. New mothers may become weepy and experience mild mood swings. These symptoms typically emerge soon after birth, peak at about 3-5 days (O'Hara, 2013) and can last a week or two. The symptoms are much milder than PPD/PPMD and usually disappear by two weeks postpartum. In most Western countries, about 80% of new mothers will have some type of mood swing after her baby is born. The birthing experience alone, whether or not it was a good experience or a bad one, can leave you emotional and weepy. All of this, coupled with sleep deprivation, fatigue, not eating well, physical discomfort, soreness or pain from the birth or from breastfeeding, and the realization that you are responsible for another human being, can all lead to postpartum or baby blues.

Symptoms may include general moodiness, mild depression, weepiness, sadness, irritability, mild anxiety, lack of concentration or feelings of dependency. The symptoms do not last long, are self-limiting and most of the time, do not need any treatment. Be aware because these symptoms can also be an early sign of depression.

General support from a loved one, a good night's sleep, joining a new mom support group or talking to other new moms or your health care provider, and eating nutritiously will do wonders for the postpartum woman experiencing postpartum blues.

Postpartum Depression

If the symptoms of the baby blues last longer than two weeks or worsen, the new mother may become diagnosed with postpartum depression and/or anxiety. Symptoms can happen gradually, or they can come on suddenly. A sudden onset of symptoms usually happens after an inflammatory response occurs, which can be triggered by some very common events of becoming a new mother, such as sleep disturbances, postpartum discomfort or pain, psychological distress, and/or trauma (Kendall-Tackett, 2007).

Sometimes symptoms can be triggered by the first menstrual cycle, or cessation of breastfeeding. Postpartum depression or anxiety can begin any time after birth and beyond the baby's first year (Bennett & Indman, 2015; Finklestein & Finklestein, 2009).

Symptoms of postpartum depression include: extreme worry, feeling irritable or in a bad mood, being short tempered, feelings of being overwhelmed, feeling very sad, feeling guilty or hopeless, developing specific phobias, sleep disturbances (either too much or too little sleep), physical symptoms, a loss of focus or concentration (frequently missing appointments), a loss of interest or pleasure in activities that used to give you joy, or a change in appetite (this can lead to either weight loss or gain). You may also feel a lack of emotional attachment towards your newborn or you may feel overly emotionally concerned and attached to your newborn.

Postpartum Anxiety Disorders

Anxiety can manifest in a few different forms, and feels very different from depression. However, the symptoms can sometimes overlap and you can have a little bit of both. Anxiety can feel like extreme nervousness, irritability, excessive worry, or fear. You may feel as if you are living on the edge, you can't cope, concentrate or focus on anything. You may have difficulty sleeping: sleeping too much or too little, or waking up during the night and not being able to fall back to sleep. You may experience either an increase or a loss of appetite, nervousness when you are with the baby, and a general feeling of being overwhelmed (Bennett & Indman, 2015). You may also experience some physical symptoms, such as stomachaches, diarrhea, nausea, vomiting, heart racing. You may feel as if you are physically ill with fatigue and/or flu like symptoms, or general aches and pains. Anxiety can also cause you to have some very upsetting thoughts and visuals. You may experience negative intrusive thoughts that you have never experienced before. As a new mother, you may become afraid to come forward and reveal to anyone that you are having these symptoms. You may become afraid that you are actually losing your mind, and you fear that your baby will be taken away from you (Beck & Driscoll, 2006; Cohen & Nonacs, 2005; Kulkarni Misri, 2005).

If you are experiencing postpartum anxiety, you may begin to experience fears that you may "snap" and harm yourself or your newborn. These type of postpartum anxiety symptoms can overlap with postpartum obsessive-compulsive disorder (POCD) (Bennett & Indman, 2015; Venis & McCloskey, 2007).

Postpartum Obsessive-Compulsive Disorder (POCD)

I had a few visuals of her in the bath and drowning her. As a result, I barely bathed her. Even now, when she takes a bath and I am sitting in the bathroom, I get nervous just remembering.

The main symptoms are the intrusive repetitive and unrelenting thoughts that were mentioned above. These thoughts are typically accompanied by behaviors to reduce the anxiety that surround them (Bennett & Indman, 2015). For example, a fear of drowning the baby in the bath would prevent you from giving the baby a bath altogether. A fear of harming the baby using a knife can result in the hiding all of the knives in the kitchen. Other repetitive behaviors can be seen, such as counting, or repeatedly checking the doors, the windows, the baby, and so on.

Gina had fears of being in her home alone with her baby when her husband traveled. She began repeatedly checking the doors to her home and was unable to stop. She went from one door to the next, checking the locks, then she started with the windows. Penny saw a bug on her baby, and began an obsessive fear of bugs, cleaning excessively and constantly checking for bugs. She saw these bugs everywhere, even if no one else did. If she saw a dot on the floor, or worse, on her baby, she would believe it was a bug. Bella saw some blood on the floor of a public restroom; her obsession with blood and blood products began. She began cleaning obsessively and became fearful to leave the house for fear that her baby will contract some disease from blood on the floor. She was cleaning to the point where she was unable to leave the house because she was never done with the checking and the cleaning.

OCD in general is a form of anxiety, and POCD can overlap with PPMD and anxiety. There may be a combination of symptoms. Scary thoughts can be a result of POCD. You may feel as if you are losing a grip on your sanity. Ruminating thoughts and excessive worry about the baby can make you feel like you are losing control. You may also have rituals of compulsively checking and rechecking the baby to make sure he is breathing, intense and unrealistic fear of germs, compulsively washing hands, or not letting anyone near the baby due to fear of germs. This syndrome can be due to a personal or family history of OCD. Some women who are experiencing a depression and anxiety may have some OCD symptoms as well (Bennett & Indman, 2015; Kleiman, 2009; Kleiman & Wenzel, 2011).

Postpartum Panic Disorder (PPPD)

I was getting my baby out of her car seat and all of a sudden I felt very sweaty, clammy, my heart started racing, and I started having chest pain. I felt like I was going to faint. It took all of my strength to get him and myself back in the car. I felt as if I was watching my body from somewhere else. It took a few minutes before I was able to calm down and drive home.

PPPD can mimic an ordinary panic attack, or general panic disorder, with the main focus of the anxiety being maternal concerns. A panic attack is a sudden rush of overpowering anxiety and fear. Your heart pounds and you feel as if you can't breathe. Some women may even feel like they are dying or going crazy. They can feel as if they are not in their own bodies and are watching themselves, as if they were on television. Panic attacks can eventually lead to panic disorder and other anxiety disorders. With postpartum panic disorder, you may fear that you are a "bad" mother, and begin to worry excessively about the baby.

These feelings of extreme anxiety and panic can come on very suddenly. You may feel physical symptoms, such as shortness of breath, chest pain, and tightness in your throat, choking sensations, dizziness and/or de-realization (an alteration in one's perception or familiarity with the outside world so that it seems unreal, like an out of body experience). You may have hot or cold flashes, sweating, trembling, restlessness, palpitations, faintness, dizziness, nausea, numbness, tingling, or loss of bodily control. The attacks may wake you up during the night, and may also come on very suddenly during the day. You begin to become so afraid of having another panic attack that you are petrified to leave the house. You may begin to withdraw from other normal activities. These attacks can be very scary, and mimic the feelings of having a heart attack. These symptoms can also overlap with postpartum posttraumatic stress disorder (PPTSD).

The panic attacks can seem to come out of nowhere and can be terrifying. You can't sleep, you are afraid to be alone, you feel as if you have no control over yourself or anything else. The cause of all this can be due to a combination of factors and is part of the release of adrenaline, also known as epinephrine, as well as the inflammatory response system. After a sudden onset of fear, a fight-or-flight response occurs, which is a bodily response to a harmful event. This disorder is sometimes seen in a woman who already has a personal or family history of anxiety and/ or panic disorder, but it can happen to any postpartum woman. These symptoms often overlap with the other postpartum anxiety related disorders. If you have experienced a difficult pregnancy or birth, your chances of developing postpartum panic disorder are greater (Bennett & Indman, 2015; Kleiman, 2009; Kleiman & Wenzel, 2011).

Postpartum Posttraumatic Stress Disorder (PPTSD)

Gabriel planned on having a natural childbirth. She read extensively and did much preparation, taking childbirth classes, practicing her breathing exercises, writing up a birth plan and organizing her home in preparation for the baby. When labor began, she and her partner headed to the hospital-based birthing center where she met with her health care team. Upon admission, her blood pressure was extremely elevated. Precautions were made, however, as her blood pressure became dangerously high, it was decided that it was best for her to undergo an emergency cesarean birth. She was placed under general anesthesia, and after the baby was born she developed HELLP (hemolysis, elevated liver enzymes, low platelet count) syndrome, a life-threatening complication of pregnancy and birth. Gabriel spent a week in the hospital, and was discharged with her baby with little support and education from her health care team.

Gabriel had a very difficult time coping immediately upon arrival at home. She had difficulty breastfeeding and was in a lot of pain from her cesarean birth. She began having flashbacks and intrusive, disturbing memories of the birth. When she did sleep, she had vivid nightmares of the birth, and was constantly worrying that something could happen to her baby. She was afraid of being alone with the baby, fearing she would "snap" and lose control.

Due to Gabriel's traumatic event, during which she felt confronted with the threat of harm to her baby, and a threat to her own physical integrity, she was diagnosed with PPTSD. Gabriel also experienced feelings of detachment and estrangement from loved ones, including her baby, hyperarousal, difficulty falling and staying asleep, and difficulty concentrating. With her symptoms of recurrent, intrusive, distressing recollections of the birth, including images, thoughts, and disturbing dreams of the birth, the diagnosis was confirmed (Zauderer, 2014).

PPTSD is a response to an extreme stressor. It is usually related to a specific trauma relating to the birth of the baby or an event from the woman's past. Some birthing mothers can experience an actual threat regarding the physical safety of themselves and/or their baby during their childbirth experience. Intense pain or a perceived or real threat of harm or death, or serious injury to themselves or their newborns, or perceived or real threatened sexual abuse can lead them to develop symptoms of PPTSD. This can occur by having the experience herself, or observing it happening to their newborn. They may respond to this trauma with feelings of intense fear, helplessness, terror, or distress. Other symptoms can include recurrent nightmares, extreme anxiety, or reliving past traumatic events. This includes sexual trauma, physical or emotional trauma, and childbirth. Women who experience a difficult or traumatic birth are at risk for having anxiety and panic attacks (Polachek, Harari, Baum, & Strous, 2012; Zauderer, 2008; 2009; 2014).

Some of the incidents that can lead to a traumatic birth and eventual PPTSD can be as follows: excessive pain, intervention by the medical staff, an unfriendly or unreceptive medical staff, a feeling of lack of control over the labor or birth, a lack of information about different procedures as they are taking place, lack of a support person, a caesarean section, a stillbirth or a sick baby. A prior risk factor for the new mother could be a history of sexual or physical abuse, a history of anxiety disorders or depression, low tolerance for pain, or a negative view of childbirth. Some women who experience this type of trauma may not develop PPTSD, but can be at risk for postpartum depression and/or anxiety (Kendall-Tackett, 2014).

A Word about Scary Thoughts

Scary thoughts are repetitive, intrusive, and unwanted thoughts that pop into your head at any given moment. Usually these thoughts will surface at the most inopportune time. These thoughts can be excessive worry, obsessing over the baby, ruminating over small things, or even having frightening images that come out of nowhere. The thoughts will not go away no matter how hard you try to get rid of them. You may have images or thoughts about accidently hurting yourself or your baby, and these images can turn into thoughts about "losing it," or "snapping," and purposely hurting your baby. *"What if I accidently drown the baby in the bathtub?" "What if I accidently drop the baby down the stairs?"* Then you may start thinking *"What if I snap or go crazy and purposely drown the baby in the bathtub?" "What if I am losing my mind and I will purposely throw the baby down the stairs?"* or *"What if I smother the baby by accident, or on purpose?" "If I think it, how do I know I won't do it?"*

These thoughts will go on and on, and may make you question your sanity. You may fear that if you told anyone about these thoughts or images, they will think you are crazy and admit you to a hospital or take your baby away from you. You are not crazy. This is not postpartum psychosis. This is anxiety. Anxiety can do some very scary things to your mind. When someone is anxious, they can have terrible thoughts about the ones that they love. Anxiety requires an outlet that expresses itself in the form of these frightening, bothersome thoughts and images. As a new mother, you love your baby so much that even if you are showing a lack of interest or not bonding with the baby, you still love him. The thought of something bad happening is so overwhelming, that your anxiety can start to play tricks on you. You then may think you are going crazy, and it just escalates from there (Kleiman & Wenzel, 2011).

What is the difference between women with scary thoughts who do not hurt anyone, and those that do?

If you are upset, or even horrified, by the thoughts you are having, you are most likely experiencing the anxiety I am speaking about. You are aware of your thoughts, and can articulate that you are having some scary thoughts and are upset by them. To actually harm your baby goes against your innate beliefs. You have the ability to distinguish right from wrong. These thoughts are not stimulated by psychosis, but by anxiety. It is highly unlikely that you will hurt anyone. Even so, because you are having so much anxiety and you are frightened, it is not a good idea for you to be alone. You should also be evaluated and treated immediately for PPMD. I usually tell new mothers that if they can sit in front of me and articulate that they are having these scary thoughts and are upset by them, it is most likely due to anxiety (Kleiman & Wenzel, 2011).

Women who harm their babies are out of touch with reality. These women are hearing voices and seeing things that are not real. These are called visual and auditory hallucinations. These women may be having serious thoughts about ending their lives and will most likely have a plan in place to do so. These women are experiencing a psychotic break, also known as postpartum psychosis (PPP), (see below) and need immediate psychiatric attention and will most likely be admitted to a facility for psychiatric treatment.

Suicidal Thoughts

Thoughts about suicide are not part of the normal PPMD experience. *Please note that regardless of what type of PPMD you have, if you are having any type of suicidal feelings, you must seek help immediately.* Suicidal thoughts are urges, sometimes voices that seem real and are heard, and a feeling that there is no way out. These thoughts can lead to a strong desire to end one's life. The desire to die is not a normal feeling, whether it is for yourself or anyone else and needs to be taken very seriously. Please tell someone if you are having these thoughts or feelings, and if they are getting stronger, let someone know immediately.

The National Suicide Prevention Lifeline at 1-800-SUICIDE is a great resource. Online, you can go to http://www.suicidepreventionlifeline.org/ and have a live chat.

If you cannot get in to see a psychiatrist or a therapist right away, you can call 911, and they will send an ambulance to take you to the nearest emergency department. If a loved one is available to take you, you can go directly to any emergency department, and there will be a psychiatrist or a psychiatric nurse practitioner on call to evaluate you. Sometimes they will send you home with medication and follow up instructions. However, if they feel that you are a danger to yourself or others, you will have to be admitted to an in-patient facility. There is no shame in doing any of the above! Your life is precious and you will get the help you need so that you can move on towards a happy and healthy life with your new family and other loved ones (American Psychological Association, 2015).

Postpartum Psychosis (PPP)

PPP is the most dangerous of all the above disorders. It is exceptionally rare, but when it happens, it is very frightening for all involved. It usually happens within the first few days or weeks after birth (Bergink, Burgerhout, Weigelt, Pop, de Wit, Drexhage, & Drexhage, 2013). PPP is known as a "psychotic break" (Blackmore, Rubinow, O'Connor, Liu, X., Tang, Craddock, & Jones, 2013; Doucet, Jones, Letourneau, Dennis, & Blackmore, 2011). Psychosis means that the new mother is not in touch with reality. The woman is very confused and is having auditory and visual delusions and hallucinations. This means that she is hearing actual voices, and seeing objects or individuals that are not really there. This should not be confused with "scary thoughts" that I talked about earlier. These women are hearing what they believe to be actual voices and seeing what they believe to be actual people.

With PPP, the woman's thoughts are irrational and disorganized, meaning that her thoughts and speech are all over the place, and she is not making any sense. These mothers have reported hearing voices in their heads telling them to do things like hurt themselves or their babies. There is often a religious theme to these voices. For example, the mother may believe that the baby is possessed, or the baby is the devil, or some other bizarre delusion. Postpartum psychosis is a psychiatric emergency and the woman needs to be hospitalized and/or treated immediately. The cause is not really known, but women with a history of bipolar disorder or schizophrenia have an increased chance of developing PPP. Treatment usually includes medication to control the hallucinations and extensive therapy. These women do recover over time, when the right treatment plan is in place (Twomey, 2009).

Pregnancy Loss or Stillbirth

The loss of a baby is a normal grieving process and not considered to be part of the PPMD continuum, however, depression, anxiety, and/or PTSD can sometimes coincide with it. The loss of a pregnancy by miscarriage or genetic termination, the loss of a newborn by stillbirth, or the birth of a child with a medical problem, a preterm birth or a congenital abnormality, can be one of the most devastating experiences that a new mother and father can undergo. These are heartbreaking events for both parents. In addition to the loss and tragic grief, you will still experience the physical symptoms of postpartum: breast tenderness, lochia bleeding, and emotional turmoil. You may struggle with grief, anxiety, guilt, and self-blame, and face more sadness than you ever thought possible. You can experience a roller coaster of emotions, such as numbness, disbelief, anger, guilt, sadness, depression, and difficulty concentrating.

Even if the pregnancy ended early on, you may have already bonded with your unborn baby. Some women can actually have physical symptoms from this emotional anguish. These symptoms include fatigue, trouble sleeping, difficulty concentrating, loss of appetite, and frequent episodes of crying. The hormonal changes that happen after the loss may increase these symptoms. Some mothers go through the normal grieving process as modeled by Elizabeth Kubler-Ross of denial, anger, bargaining, depression, and, at last, acceptance.

Diagnosis

Professionals specializing in PPMD are trained to assess the new mother based on the current symptoms, personal and family history, support system, and pregnancy and birthing experience. In addition, there are many tools or questionnaires that help the clinician gather information in order to form a diagnosis. You may be given a questionnaire to fill out during your visit, which will then be discussed with you regarding the results. The two most common questionnaires are the PDSS Postpartum Depression Screening Scale by Beck and Gable, which is a 35-question self-report scale (Beck & Driscoll, 2006), and the EPDS (Edinburgh

Postnatal Depression Scale,) which is a 10-question screening scale (example shown at the end of this chapter).

It is also important to get a full medical workup if you are not feeling like yourself, as there are a number of physiological imbalances that can offset some of the symptoms of depression and anxiety. For example, hypothyroidism can cause depression, and hyperthyroidism can cause anxiety.

Treatment

As a new mother, you may be afraid to take the first steps toward seeing a professional. Just because you seek professional care does not mean that you are going "crazy." The same way you would seek help from a specialist if you had a thyroid problem or a blood-sugar problem, you need to be screened for PPMD. The most important thing is that you recover and get back to yourself as soon as possible. Getting prompt treatment will prevent the symptoms from worsening, which can then become more difficult to treat (Bennett & Indman, 2015).

Finding the right professional can be tricky, and it is important to see someone who is familiar with, or even specializes in PPMD. There are many postpartum websites where you can find a professional who specializes in treating PPMD. Postpartum Support International (PSI), http://www.postpartum.net/ is a great resource where you can find important information on PPMD, local resources, such as clinicians in your area, or support groups, chat rooms and a tremendous amount of other information. There is also The Marce Society http://marcesociety.com/, http://www.postpartumhealthalliance.org/, and North American Society for Psychosocial OB/GYN, http://www.naspog.org/website/. There are also many blogs for new mothers where they can interact with other mothers or gain access to valuable information, such as Postpartum Progress http://www.postpartumprogress.com/.

As recognition of PPMD increases, many states provide local postpartum organizations that can offer referrals and other services. Professionals would include a clinical social worker, psychologist, or clinical nurse specialist who provides psychotherapy, which is talk therapy. Psychiatrists or psychiatric nurse practitioners, provide both therapy and medication management. Other connections for you to make can be anyone with whom you feel comfortable, such as your OB/GYN, nurse-midwife, pediatrician, lactation consultant, faith-community member, family member, doula, or a phone volunteer.

Treatment for PPMD uses a holistic approach. It focuses on what you need medically, mentally, and emotionally in order to make a complete recovery. It is a combination of psychotherapy, social support, and possibly medication. Talk therapy would include crisis management. The focus is on ways to reduce the symptoms, and help you to reorganize your life to get the help you need so you can rest, eat, sleep, and recover. You need to remind yourself that you will recover, you are not alone, and this is not your fault. You are a good mother, and you need to take care of yourself in order to take care of your family. You are doing the best that you can.

Restoring balance to the new mother is crucial. Sleeping and eating are basics. A healthy diet is very important for your recovery. You may not have an appetite, however, it is important to push yourself to eat. Some women will eat too much or consume junk food. Protein, water, protein shakes, fruits, vegetables, and whole grains are good foods to eat while avoiding caffeine (especially if you are having anxiety), sugar, and carbohydrates. Activity is important. Brisk physical exercise can raise endorphin levels and help elevate your mood. Taking breaks and getting regular scheduled time off from duties surrounding the baby and household responsibilities, as well as getting outside for fresh air and sunshine both promote recovery (Ellsworth-Bowers & Corwin, 2012; Zauderer & Davis, 2012).

Do not be afraid to ask for help. Having a good support system: partner, family, extended family, neighbors, co-workers, religious communities, doulas, nannies, lactation consultants, housekeepers, hotlines, support groups, and chat rooms, are all helpful for a complete recovery. If you are dealing with anxiety or obsessions, in addition to avoiding caffeine, it is advisable to avoid television news and newspapers. Reading or watching other people's tragedies might cause you to absorb it into your own life and can increase your anxiety. Journaling feelings and reading some self-help books can also help with recovery (Raymond, Pratt, Godecker, Harrison, Kim, Kuendig, & O'Brien, 2014). Some books about PPMD may be too upsetting for you to read; therefore, this should be done via the recommendation of your clinician.

There are many natural supplements that can be used for treatment. Make sure to take these with the guidance of a clinician, as some herbs and supplements have not yet been FDA approved. Even though these products are natural, they may have some side effects. Some supplements that can help with PPMD symptoms are Omega-3 fatty acids and Fish Oil. Vitamin B complex, Vitamin C, Calcium, Magnesium, and Iron, can also be helpful in relieving some of these symptoms. Some herbs commonly used to treat PPMD are Ginseng, Ginko Gilboa, Sam-e, and St. Johns Wort. Some herbal teas contain these ingredients and can have a calming effect such as: St. Johns Wort, Valerian, and Chamomile (Bennett, & Indman, 2015; Zauderer & Davis, 2012).

If you are concerned about breastfeeding and taking medication or herbal supplements, there are a number of websites where you can look up information or even to speak to a specialist in *teratology*. Teratology is a branch of medicine that focuses on physical abnormalities of the fetus during pregnancy and breastfeeding. There are a number of organizations of specialists who respond to the public about concerns regarding any type of exposure during pregnancy or breastfeeding such as Lactmed https://www.data.gov/applications/lactmed/. There is also Infant Risk Center (IRC) infantrisk.org, or MommyMeds.com (MM). The InfantRisk Center also has an app for smart phones called Mommy Meds designed for use by new mothers. IRC and MM support the research of Dr. Thomas Hale, a clinical pharmacologist, and an expert in the use of medications and breastfeeding. He is also the author of the book *Medications and Mothers' Milk* (2014).

Another natural remedy that has been found to be helpful is bright light therapy—either 20 to 30 minutes of an artificial therapy light. Bright light therapy has been proven to be extremely effective in treating many different types of depression. It is a good option in the treatment of PPMD since it is cost effective, can be used in the home, and may not have the side effects of some of the medications used to treat PPMD (Crowley & Youngstedt, 2012). Massage therapy, acupuncture, yoga, regular exercise, meditation and/or relaxation exercises or tapes can also help to lift your spirits, calm you down and restore and balance your mood (Deligiannidis & Freeman, 2014).

Medication

All of these natural remedies can be used to treat PMD. However, you should not be afraid to take medication if you are not improving, and if your clinician feels that you would benefit from it. Medications can be used together with many holistic treatments (except for the herbal supplements). Many women fear these medications will turn them into "zombies" or have uncontrollable side effects. Others fear the old-fashioned stigma attached to some medications and that they will be labeled as "crazy." The psychiatric medications used today to treat PPMD are very mild, the dose is adjusted so that you will improve without feeling like a "zombie," and they have mild side effects. Treating PPMD symptoms is as important as treating any other medical condition, such as high blood pressure, diabetes, or asthma (Hale & Rowe, 2014).

A new mother suffering from PPMD who wishes to breastfeed is often faced with a difficult decision. Gather as much information as you can. Should I take medication and breastfeed? Continue to breastfeed and forgo the medication? Or discontinue breastfeeding so that I can take the medication and not have to worry about the effects on my baby? These questions all come into play when making this decision and it is a very personal choice. You can also try CAM (complementary and alternative medicine) treatments, as mentioned above. It is important to remember that the baby will be exposed to either the medication or the depression if left untreated. If you choose to take the medication, or even CAM and continue to breastfeed, you should find a pediatric health care provider that fully supports your decision. Studies have shown that there is a very low risk in most of the medications used to treat PPMD and discussing them with a medical provider or pediatric team can be very helpful in making that decision (Zauderer & Galea, 2010).

The most common medications used in the treatment of PPMD, and the first-line of treatment is selective serotonin-reuptake inhibitors (SSRI). These medications increase serotonin, which is known as your "feel good" hormone, or neurotransmitter. These medications usually take about two to six weeks for the full effect to take place. Some women feel good after only a couple of days and for some women, it can take the full six weeks for them to feel better. These medications are used for both anxiety and depression. They generally work very well and have fewer side effects than other classes of antidepressant/antianxiety medications. Some of the side effects that may be experienced are mild nausea, diarrhea, headache, sweating, bad dreams or very vivid dreams, dizziness, dry mouth, or sexual dysfunction. Most of the side effects go away within the first few weeks except for the dry mouth and sexual side effects, which may last for the duration that one is on the medication (Bennet, 2009; Bennett & Indman, 2015; Dowd Stone & Menken, 2008; Hale & Rowe, 2014).

The most commonly used medications are: Prozac (fluoxetine), Zoloft (sertraline), Paxil (paroxetine), Celexa (citalopram), Lexapro (escitalopram), and Luvox (fluvoxamine). Paxil is contraindicated during pregnancy, but can be used during breastfeeding. Another group of medications are called the serotonin-norepinephrine reuptake inhibitors (SNRI). These include Effexor (venlafaxine), Cymbalta (duloxetine) and Pristiq (desvenlafaxine). Wellbutrin (buproprion), which is norepinephrine-dopamine reuptake inhibitor (NDRI), and Remeron a noradrenergic and specific serotonergic antidepressant (NaSSA), may be considered if the other medications are not working well, or in addition to other medications.

According to the experts in the field, Dr. Thomas Hale, InfantRisk, and LactMed, the preferred medications during pregnancy and breastfeeding are Prozac (fluoxetine), Zoloft (sertraline), and Lexapro (escitalopram citalopram).

If you are having extreme anxiety and panic and your medication has not yet taken effect, you may be offered a class of anti-anxiety medication called benzodiazepines. These are commonly known as mild tranquilizers. These medications will offer you immediate relief of your anxiety in order for you to be able to function until the SSRIs or antidepressants/antianxiety medications take effect. They are also highly addictive so they should only be used for a very short amount of time, or once in a while for situational anxiety.

These medications include Xanax (alprazolam), Ativan (lorazepam) which are short acting and leave the body after a few hours, Valium (diazepam) and Klonopin (clonazepam), which take longer to leave the body. These medications should be used with caution while breastfeeding, with your pediatric health care providers' approval (Iqbal, Sobhan, & Ryals, 2014; Noble, 2012). For much more severe cases of PPMD or postpartum psychosis, the clinician may use mood stabilizers, sleep aids, antipsychotics, and sometimes electroconvulsive therapy (ECT) (Bennett & Indman, 2015; Twomey, 2009).

If you are having symptoms or you know of anyone who is having symptoms, please do not keep this to yourself. Please share your concerns with a loved one or a health care professional. PPMD is nothing to be ashamed of and help is readily available if you seek it. Early detection and treatment will help you get the help you need so that you will be able to pull yourself out of this fog. Please don't be resistant to treatment. Take the right steps to feel good again, so that you can become the mother that you were meant to be.

"I didn't know how badly I was feeling, until I started to feel good again"

Resources

American Psychiatric Association (APA)

1000 Wilson Boulevard, Suite 182
Arlington, VA 22209
www.psych.org
email: apa@psych.org
Call Toll-Free: 1-888-35-PSYCH
or 1-888-35-77924
From outside the U.S. and Canada
call: 1-703-907-7300

American Psychological Association (APA)

750 First Street NE
Washington DC, 20002-4242
www.apa.org
800-374-2721

National Institute of Mental Health (NIMH)

www.nimh.nih.gov
email: nimhinfo@nih.gov
1-866-615-6464 (toll-free)
1-301-443-8431 (TTY)
1-866-415-8051 (TTY toll-free)

North Shore University Health Systems: Jennifer's story

http://www.northshore.org/maternal-health/before-and-after-delivery/perinatal-depression/jennifers-story/
Support Line: 866-364-MOMS (6667)

Postpartum Men

5835 College Avenue, Suite D3
Oakland, Ca. 94618
Postpartummen.com
415-346-6719

Postpartum Progress (blog)

www.postpartumprogress.com

Postpartum Resource Center of New York Inc. (PRC)

109 Udall Road
West Islip, NY 11795
www.postpartumny.org
631-422-2255
Toll Free-855-631-0001

Postpartum Support International (PSI)

6706 SW 54th Avenue
Portland, Oregon 97219 USA
www.postpartum.net
email: support@postpartum.net
PSI Office Telephone: 503-894-9453 | Fax: 503-894-9452
Support Helpline: 800.944.4PPD (4773)

The Postpartum Stress Center LLC

1062 Lancaster Avenue, Rosemont Plaza, Suite 2
Rosemont, Pennsylvania 19010
610.525.7527
151 Fries Mill Road, Suite 201
Turnersville, New Jersey 08012
856.302.1381
www.postpartumstress.com
email: info@postpartumstress.com

LactMed

http://toxnet.nlm.nih.gov/cgi-bin/sis/htmlgen?LACTMED

InfantRisk

http://www.infantrisk.com/

Chapter 10
Post-Baby Bonding and Attachment: Enjoying Your Baby

"What does bonding and attachment mean?"
"Am I supposed to bond or attach with my baby right away?"
"What can I do to form a bond or attachment?"

Bonding occurs when you and your newborn form a strong connection to each other beginning the moment you lay eyes on her. You will feel a tremendous amount of joy when you are with your newborn, and a strong desire to protect her. A bond is your baby's first relationship with someone. It provides security and helps her to learn about trust. A secure attachment will help your baby form trusting, strong relationships with others as they get older.

Attachment is an ongoing process; it may begin during pregnancy, or later on, but it continues throughout our lives. Attachment with a new individual follows a natural progression, but it may not happen right away and is not always automatic. You may have formed an attachment with your newborn ever since the moment you found out that you were expecting. Or it may take a few days, weeks, or possibly even months after birth. Don't feel badly if you have not felt this attachment yet, as it has no reflection on you or your parenting. It is a gradual process, and you may not even know it is happening. Keep on taking good care of your newborn, respond to her needs, and your attachment will develop. Learn ways to calm your newborn. When you feel you can soothe her, your feelings of attachment will deepen. Your maternal instincts will begin to shine through at some point very soon. Be patient: it will happen and it will be wonderful.

There are several reasons why you may not have bonded with your newborn immediately:

- ▸ You experienced a difficult or traumatic childbirth.
- ▸ You had an unexpected cesarean birth or any type of assisted vaginal delivery, such as forceps or vacuum birth, and you are still in pain.
- ▸ Your newborn spent time in the Neonatal Intensive Care Unit.
- ▸ Your newborn was, or is, in need of medical treatments or procedures.
- ▸ You had a difficult time conceiving, experienced fertility treatments, adopted, or used donor eggs or sperm.
- ▸ You are experiencing a postpartum/perinatal mood disorder.

How Can I Form An Attachment When All My Baby Does Is Cry?

Bringing home a new baby can be one of the most rewarding, yet challenging times for you, as a new mother. Caring for a newborn is a 24/7 job. Accepting that, in the beginning, life will be hectic and crazy will help you cope better. As long as all your newborn's basic needs are met, she is fed, burped, clean, and dry, nothing is sticking or hurting her, she is not too hot or too cold, and nothing is medically wrong (such as a fever), she may just need to be held, and rocked. She may still cry while you are doing this, but a newborn should not be left to cry alone. Try to comfort her as best as you can, but she still may cry in your arms. Some newborn babies are colicky, and you should discuss excessive crying with your pediatric health care provider. If this is the case, you may need to change your formula (if bottle feeding), or possibly eliminate some gas producing foods from your diet that can be causing the discomfort (if you are breastfeeding). You need not go to extremes with your diet, as sometimes eliminating foods does not help with preventing baby's gas. Sometimes babies just need to fuss and cry.

Your newborn may be releasing some emotions from the trauma of her birth through crying. Some babies have a particular time of the day that they fuss or cry, and you will find that they tend to cry during that same time every day. During the rest of the day or night, they may be fine. For some newborns, their fussy time may be for an hour or two (if your newborn fusses longer than that, you may want to ask your pediatric health care provider about it). Just be happy if it is not in the middle of the night. Some babies like to be held and will start to cry when you put them down. You can find creative ways to carry your newborn, and remember, you are not spoiling her by carrying her. Your newborn is much too young to understand the art of manipulation—she is communicating with you. Let your newborn know you are there for her. She will grow up to feel more secure knowing that you were there for her when she needed you.

Colic, general crying, and fussing will usually subside by the time your baby is 3 months old. I know that this seems like a long time, and it can become very frustrating to try and soothe an inconsolable baby. Do the best you can, and know that it will stop. If you can get someone to help and give you a break once in a while, that would be very beneficial.

Things you can do for a fussy newborn:

- Keep them in motion: rocking, carrying, and moving.
- Keep them close to you.
- Dance to music.
- Go for a walk with the stroller.
- Swaddle.
- Practice skin to skin.
- Go for a car ride.
- Play white noise from a noise machine, or use a vacuum cleaner or hair dryer.
- Try infant massage, which can help them to relieve some gas.
- Try herbal remedies, but ask your pediatric health care provider first.
- Avoid letting your newborn "cry it out" in her crib or bassinet. No one likes to cry alone.

I thought I went deaf, I woke up one morning and didn't hear crying, I had a happy baby, her whole demeanor changed. It was wonderful!

The Bonding and Attachment Process

Not all new mothers bond with their babies as soon as they are born. You may melt the minute you see her and instantly fall in love, feeling emotions you never knew you had. Or after a very difficult birth, you may feel disappointed, or feel nothing at all except pain and discomfort. The attachment process is different for every new mother or father, and will grow and develop throughout your baby's lifetime. Don't feel as if you missed a golden opportunity to form an attachment if you did not feel instantaneous bonding with your newborn. You will need time to heal physically and emotionally and to get used to the fact that you are a mother.

How Can I Help the Bonding-Attachment Process?

Nourish and take care of yourself. If you are healthy, you will have an easier time and more patience to attach to your newborn. Your newborn is very sensitive to smell. So for the first few weeks, don't confuse your newborn by wearing perfume or scented deodorants, as you want her to get used to your own natural scent (U.S. Department of Health & Human Services, 2013). Other ways to encourage secure attachment are:

- ▸ Practice skin-to-skin contact.
- ▸ Hold your newborn close when feeding, whether breast or bottle.
- ▸ Hold your newborn close when comforting.
- ▸ Respond to her cries.
- ▸ Talk, smile, laugh, read, and sing to your newborn.
- ▸ Make a lot of eye contact.
- ▸ Dance with your newborn to music you like.
- ▸ Instead of using the swing, rocker, or other baby paraphernalia,

which keep your newborn away from you, wear your newborn instead, keeping them close to you (such as in a sling, snuggly, etc.).

How Can Dad Attach?

- ▸ Burp, bathe, diaper, and comfort your newborn.
- ▸ Spend time with her without mom.
- ▸ Practice skin-to-skin contact.
- ▸ Feed formula or pumped milk in a bottle.
- ▸ Wear your newborn in a sling or snuggly.

Seek professional help if, after 6 to 8 weeks, you feel resentful, disconnected, or indifferent to your baby, have not bonded at all yet, or if you are experiencing signs and symptoms of a postpartum or perinatal mood disorder (PPMD) (see Chapter 9).

Enjoying your Baby

As your baby gets older, you can find plenty of opportunities for interaction and have a lot of fun with her. Getting out to some local groups and activities will not only help the two of you develop a secure attachment, but also will be good socialization for both you and baby. Many new mothers meet lifelong friends in their mommy classes, and their children often grow up together.

- ▸ Play, play, play with your baby (if you don't know how, learn).
- ▸ Join a mommy-and-me or a Gymboree class where you can learn interactive songs and activities (like "the wheels on the bus").
- ▸ Get videos out from the library, or stream from YouTube or Netflix, which you can sing to and watch together.
- ▸ Bring your baby to the library or local bookstore for story hour.
- ▸ Read books. Point out objects, animals, and colors.
- ▸ Go for long walks.

- ► Go to a park on a nice day. You can bring a book with you if your baby naps, this is a good opportunity to meet other new mothers.

- ► As your baby gets older, you can go to a zoo or a children's museum.

- ►"Fit4mom" is a stroller-based fitness program for mothers and babies, and is a great way to get in shape, learn interactive play with your baby, and meet other new moms.

Lose Yourself in Motherhood, But Don't Forget Who You Are

The first 6 weeks after childbirth is all about protecting and nurturing your newborn. Your baby needs you now more than she ever will again. The first 6 weeks are difficult, and you may feel isolated and trapped. There is a fine line between embracing motherhood and nourishing yourself as an individual. It's very hard, but it's worth it.

For now, it is okay to lose yourself in motherhood, but don't forget who you are and the things you love. Remember your hobbies, talents, and career. You may be a singer, songwriter, artist, painter, dancer, runner, or swimmer. Don't give up on your dreams. It may be a little harder now, but your children will grow up to see you as a talented person, respect who you are, and learn from you. Children learn best by observation. Your children will become like you and follow their dreams when they see you following yours. This is not as easy as it seems, as your priorities change and family does come first.

A mother who feels good about herself will raise children who feel good about themselves. This doesn't mean you have to go back to work. If you chose to be a stay-at-home mom, you can nourish your soul and develop your inner self in other ways. Be creative and use your talents to fulfill your creative needs, or you might feel resentful later on. You may have to alter your dreams a little bit—for instance, instead of being a concert pianist, you may settle for playing at local shows, at home for yourself or your children, or teaching music in a school.

Don't make your children's life your life. It is not good for your self-esteem and might make your child feel overpowered by you. Allow your children the space to explore their own dreams and talents, not yours. Let them find their own path and don't live your dreams vicariously through them. Confident women will raise confident children, and mentally healthy woman will give children the confidence and ability to be mentally healthy as well.

Becoming a Mother

Motherhood is one of the greatest joys in life, and probably the best thing that will ever happen to you. You can't give your newborn too much love. Study and learn about babies' basic care from books, friends who are parents, your own parents, and your pediatric health care provider. After you ask or receive advice from others, go ahead and trust your own instincts.

The best advice I ever received was "don't listen to anyone."

Discover who you are as a mother. Motherhood can be extremely rewarding. However, parenthood, in general, consists of many highs and lows. Your newborn may cry for 3 months straight. But when she smiles at you for the first time (*really* smiles, not just gas), you will feel that it was all worth it. Baby's first steps, first words, first day of school, first graduation, and all the other milestones you have before you will bring you so much joy that the hardships in between will be outshined by them. Remind yourself of these moments when you are struggling or having a rough day. Motherhood is the most demanding job on the planet. It is a path on a larger journey that brings many surprises and rewards.

Resources

Fit4mom

http://fit4mom.com/

Gymboree

http://www.gymboreeclasses.com/en/

Mommy & Me

http://www.mommyandme.com/

Parents.com

http://www.parents.com/baby/new-parent/motherhood/fun-things-to-do-with-your-baby/

References

Academy of Breastfeeding Medicine (ABM) Protocol. (2010). ABM clinical protocol# 8: human milk storage information for home use for full-term infants (original protocol March 2004; revision# 1 March 2010). *Breastfeeding Medicine, 5*(3), 127-130.

Ahmadi, F., Siahbazi, S., & Akhbari, F. (2013). Incomplete cesarean scar rupture. *Journal of Reproduction & Infertility, 14*(1), 43.

Allen, L. H. (2012). B vitamins in breast milk: relative importance of maternal status and intake, and effects on infant status and function. *Advances in Nutrition: An International Review Journal, 3*(3), 362-369.

American Academy of Pediatrics (AAP). (2015). *Amount and schedule of formula feedings.* Retrieved from http://www.healthychildren.org/English/ages-stages/baby/feeding-nutrition/Pages/Amount-and-Schedule-of-Formula-Feedings.aspx

American Academy of Pediatrics. (2012). *AAP reaffirms breastfeeding guidelines.* http://www.aap .org/en-us/about-the-aap/aap-press-room/pages/AAP-Reaffirms-Breastfeeding-Guidelines.aspx

American Psychological Association. (2015). *Postpartum depression.* http://www.apa.org/pi/women/programs/depression/ postpartum.aspx, (2015).

Audelo, L. (2013). *The virtual breastfeeding culture: Seeking mother-to-mother support in the digital age.* Amarillo, TX: Praeclarus Press.

Bartz, J. A., Zaki, J., Bolger, N., & Ochsner, K. N. (2011). Social effects of oxytocin in humans: Context and person matter. *Trends in Cognitive Sciences, 15*(7), 301-309.

Beck, C.T., & Driscoll, J.W. (2006). *Postpartum mood and anxiety disorders: A clinician's guide.* Sudbury, MA: Jones and Bartlett.

Benefer, M., Corfe, B., Russell, J., Short, R., & Barker, M. (2013). Water intake and post-exercise cognitive performance: An observational study of long-distance walkers and runners. *European Journal of Nutrition, 52*(2), 617-624.

Bennett, S.S. (2009). *Pregnant on Prozac: The essential guide to making the best decision for you and your baby.* Guilford, CT: The Globe Pequot Press.

Bennett, S., & Indman, P. (2015). *Beyond the blues: Understanding and treating prenatal and postpartum depression & anxiety.* San Francisco, CA: Untreed Reads Publishing.

Bergink, V., Burgerhout, K. M., Weigelt, K., Pop, V. J., de Wit, H., Drexhage, R. C., ... & Drexhage, H. A. (2013). Immune system dysregulation in first-onset postpartum psychosis. *Biological Psychiatry, 73*(10), 1000-1007.

Blackmore, E. R., Rubinow, D. R., O'Connor, T. G., Liu, X., Tang, W., Craddock, N., & Jones, I. (2013). Reproductive outcomes and risk of subsequent illness in women diagnosed with postpartum psychosis. *Bipolar Disorders, 15*(4), 394-404.

Birth control methods fact sheet. (2012). http://www.womenshealth.gov/publications/our-publications/fact-sheet/birth-control-methods.html

Bonanno, C., Clausing, M., & Berkowitz, R. (2011). VBAC: A medicolegal perspective. *Clinics in Perinatology, 38*(2), 217-225.

Brenner, M. G., & Buescher, E. S. (2011). Breastfeeding: A clinical imperative. *Journal of Women's Health, 20*(12), 1767-1773.

Briggs, G. G., Freeman, R. K., & Yaffe, S. J. (2012). *Drugs in pregnancy and lactation: A reference guide to fetal and neonatal risk.* Philadelphia, PA: Lippincott Williams & Wilkins.

Brizendine, L. (2006). *The female brain.* New York: Morgan Road Books.

Brunton, P. J., Russell, J. A., & Hirst, J. J. (2014). Allopregnanolone in the brain: Protecting pregnancy and birth outcomes. *Progress in Neurobiology, 113,* 106-136.

Buttner, M. M., O'Hara, M. W., & Watson, D. (2012). The structure of women's mood in the early postpartum. *Assessment, 19*(2), 247-256.

Cohen, L.S., & Nonacs, R.M. (2005). *Mood and anxiety disorders during pregnancy and postpartum.* Washington, DC: American Psychiatric Publishing.

Colson, S. (2005). Maternal breastfeeding positions: Have we got it right? (2). *The Practising Midwife, 8*(11), 29-32.

Colson, S.D. (2012). *Biological nurturing.* Retrieved from: http://www.biologicalnurturing.com/pages/ philosophy.html.

Cong, X., Ludington-Hoe, S. M., Hussain, N., Cusson, R. M., Walsh, S., Vazquez, V., Briere, C.E., & Vittner, D. (2015). Parental oxytocin responses during skin-to-skin contact in pre-term infants. *Early Human Development, 91*(7), 401-406.

Cotterman, K. J. (2004). Reverse pressure softening: A simple tool to prepare areola for easier latching during engorgement. *Journal of Human Lactation, 20*(2), 227-237.

Crowley, S. K., & Youngstedt, S. D. (2012). Efficacy of light therapy for perinatal depression: A review. *Journal of Physiological Anthropology, 31*(1), 15-15.

Daley, A. J., Thomas, A., Cooper, H., Fitzpatrick, H., McDonald, C., Moore, H., & Deeks, J. J. (2012). Maternal exercise and growth in breastfed infants: A meta-analysis of randomized controlled trials. *Pediatrics, 130*(1), 108-114.

Davanzo, R., De Cunto, A., Paviotti, G., Travan, L., Inglese, S., Brovedani, P., & Demarini, S. (2014). Making the first days of life safer preventing Sudden Unexpected Postnatal Collapse while promoting breastfeeding. *Journal of Human Lactation, 31*, 12-14

Deligiannidis, K. M., & Freeman, M. P. (2014). Complementary and alternative medicine therapies for perinatal depression. *Best Practice & Research Clinical Obstetrics & Gynaecology, 28*(1), 85-95.

Doucet, S., Jones, I., Letourneau, N., Dennis, C. L., & Blackmore, E. R. (2011). Interventions for the prevention and treatment of postpartum psychosis: A systematic review. *Archives of Women's Mental Health, 14*(2), 89-98.

Dowd Stone, S., & Menken, A.E. (2008). *Perinatal and postpartum mood disorders: Perspectives and treatment guide for the health care practitioner.* New York: Springer Publishing Company.

Duggan, C., Srinivasan, K., Thomas, T., Samuel, T., Rajendran, R., Muthayya, S., & Kurpad, A. V. (2014). Vitamin B-12 supplementation during pregnancy and early lactation increases maternal, breast milk, and infant measures of vitamin B-12 status. *Journal of Nutrition, 144*(5), 758-764.

Durante, K. M., Griskevicius, V., Simpson, J. A., Cantú, S. M., & Tybur, J. M. (2012). Sex ratio and women's career choice: Does a scarcity of men lead women to choose briefcase over baby? *Journal of Personality and Social Psychology, 103*(1), 1-15

Durham, R., & Chapman, L. (2014). Postpartal period. In *Maternal-newborn nursing: The critical components of nursing care, 2nd Ed.*(pp. 309-335). Philadelphia: F.A. Davis.

Eden, K. B., Denman, M. A., Emeis, C. L., McDonagh, M. S., Fu, R., Janik, R. K., & Guise, J. M. (2012). Trial of labor and vaginal delivery rates in women with a prior cesarean. *Journal of Obstetric, Gynecologic, & Neonatal Nursing, 41*(5), 583-598.

Eidelman, A. I., Schanler, R. J., Johnston, M., Landers, S., Noble, L., Szucs, K., & Viehmann, L. (2012). Breastfeeding and the use of human milk. *Pediatrics, 129*(3), e827-e841.

Elliot-Carter, N. E. V. A., & Harper, J. (2012). Keeping mothers and newborns together after cesarean. *Nursing for Women's Health, 16*(4), 290-295.

Ellsworth-Bowers, E. R., & Corwin, E. J. (2012). Nutrition and the psychoneuroimmunology of postpartum depression. *Nutrition Research Reviews, 25*(01), 180-192.

Farr, S. A., Price, T. O., Dominguez, L. J., Motisi, A., Saiano, F., Niehoff, M. L., & Barbagallo, M. (2012). Extra virgin olive oil improves learning and memory in SAMP8 mice. *Journal of Alzheimer's Disease, 28*(1), 81-92.

Finklestein, B., & Finklestein, M. (2009). *Delivery from darkness: A Jewish guide to prevention and treatment of postpartum depression.* New York: Feldheim.

Fletcher, G. J., Simpson, J. A., Campbell, L., & Overall, N. C. (2015). Pair-bonding, romantic love, and evolution: The curious case of homosapiens. *Perspectives on Psychological Science, 10*(1), 20-36.

Ganzer, C. A., & Zauderer, C. R. (2011). Promoting a brain-healthy lifestyle: Simple adjustments to diet, exercise and social and cognitive stimulation, can slow the effects of ageing on the brain. *Nursing Older People, 23*(7), 24-27.

Gartner, L. M., Morton, J., Lawrence, R. A., Naylor, A. J., O'Hare, D., Schanler, R. J., & Eidelman, A. I. (2005). Breastfeeding and the use of human milk. *Pediatrics, 115*(2), 496-506.

Gouchon, S., Gregori, D., Picotto, A., Patrucco, G., Nangeroni, M., & Di Giulio, P. (2010). Skin-to-skin contact after cesarean delivery: An experimental study. *Nursing Research, 59*(2), 78-84.

Gray, R. H., Campbell, O. M., Apelo, R., Eslami, S. S., Zacur, H., Ramos, R. M., & Labbok, M. H. (1990). Risk of ovulation during lactation. *The Lancet, 335*(8680), 25-29.

Graziano, S., Murphy, D., Braginsky, L., Horwitz, J., Kennedy, V., Burkett, D., & Kenton, K. (2014). Assessment of bowel function in the peripartum period. *Archives of Gynecology and Obstetrics, 289*(1), 23-27.

Guise, J. M., Denman, M. A., Emeis, C., Marshall, N., Walker, M., Fu, R., & McDonagh, M. (2010). Vaginal birth after cesarean: New insights on maternal and neonatal outcomes. *Obstetrics & Gynecology, 115*(6), 1267-1278.

Hale, T. W., & Rowe, H. E. (2014). *Medications and mothers' milk, 16th. Ed.* Plano, TX: Hale Publishing.

Henderson, A. (2011). Understanding the breast crawl. *Nursing for Women's Health, 15*(4), 296-307.

Hoffman, S. A., Massett, S. K., & Sorber, J. L. (2014). Supporting kangaroo care after cesarean birth: Going bare for better care. *Journal of Obstetric, Gynecologic, & Neonatal Nursing, 43*(S1), S60.

Hung, K. J., & Berg, O. (2011). Early skin-to-skin after cesarean to improve breastfeeding. *MCN: The American Journal of Maternal/Child Nursing, 36*(5), 318-324.

Hunter, T., & Cattelona, G. (2014). Breastfeeding initiation and duration in first-time mothers: Exploring the impact of father involvement in the early post-partum period. *Health Promotion Perspectives, 4*(2), 132-136.

Iqbal, M. M., Sobhan, T., & Ryals, T. (2014). Effects of commonly used benzo-diazepines on the fetus, the neonate, and the nursing infant. *Psychiatric Services, 53*(1), 39-49.

Johnson, E., Vishwanathan, R., Mohn, E., Haddock, J., Rasmussen, H., & Scott, T. (2015). Avocado consumption increases neural lutein and improves cognitive function. *The FASEB Journal, 29*(1 Supplement), 32-38.

Jones, A. D., Ickes, S. B., Smith, L. E., Mduduzi, M. N., Chasekwa, B., Heid-kamp, R. A., & Stoltzfus, R. J. (2013). World Health Organization infant and young child feeding indicators and their associations with child growth: A synthesis of recent findings. *The FASEB Journal, 27*, 618-612.

Kendall-Tackett, K. (2014). Childbirth-related posttraumatic stress disorder: Symptoms and impact on breastfeeding. *Clinical Lactation, 5*(2), 51-55.

Kendall-Tackett, K. (2007). A new paradigm for depression in new mothers: The central role of inflammation and how breastfeeding and anti-in-flammatory treatments protect maternal mental health. *International Breastfeeding Journal, 2*(6), 19.

Kim, P., Leckman, J. F., Mayes, L. C., Feldman, R., Wang, X., & Swain, J. E. (2010). The plasticity of human maternal brain: Longitudinal changes in brain anatomy during the early postpartum period. *Behavioral Neuro-science, 124*(5), 695.

Kleiman, K., & Wenzel, A. (2014). *Tokens of affection: Reclaiming your marriage after postpartum depression.* New York: Routledge.

Kleiman, K., & Wenzel, A. (2011). *Dropping the baby and other scary thoughts: Breaking the cycle of unwanted thoughts in motherhood.* New York: Routledge.

Kotila, L. E., & Kamp Dush, C. M. (2012). Another baby? Father involvement and childbearing in fragile families. *Journal of Family Psychology, 26*(6), 976-986.

Krikorian, R., Shidler, M. D., Nash, T. A., Kalt, W., Vinqvist-Tymchuk, M. R., Shukitt-Hale, B., & Joseph, J. A. (2010). Blueberry supplementation improves memory in older adults†. *Journal of Agricultural and Food Chemistry, 58*(7), 3996-4000.

Kulkarni Misri, S. (2005). *Pregnancy blues: What every woman needs to know about depression during pregnancy.* New York: Bantam Dell.

Kuyper, E., Vitta, B., & Dewey, K. (2014). Implications of cesarean delivery for breastfeeding outcomes and strategies to support breastfeeding. *Insight, 8*, 1-9.

Labbok, M. (2008). Exploration of guilt among mothers who do not breast-feed: The physician's role. *Journal of Human Lactation, 24*(1), 80-84.

Lamaze International (2014). *A woman's guide to VBAC: Navigating the NIH Consensus Recommendations.* http://www.givingbirthwithconfidence.org/p/bl/et/blogid=16&blogaid=933

Lawrence, R. A., & Lawrence, R. M. (2010). *Breastfeeding: A guide for the medical professional, 7th Ed.* New York: Elsevier Saunders.

Lim, R., Barnett-Lopez, M., & Franciso, J. (2004). *After the baby's birth: A complete guide for postpartum women.* Berkeley, CA: Celestial Arts.

Lowdermilk, D. L., Perry, S. E., & Cashion, M. C. (2014). Nursing care of the family during the postpartum period. In *Maternity Nursing-Revised*, 8*th* Ed. (pp. 481-501). Maryland Heights, MO: Elsevier Health Sciences.

Ludington-Hoe, S. M., & Morgan, K. (2014). Infant assessment and reduction of sudden unexpected postnatal collapse risk during skin-to-skin contact. *Newborn and Infant Nursing Reviews, 14*(1), 28-33.

Lundgren, I., Begley, C., Gross, M. M., & Bondas, T. (2012). 'Groping through the fog': A metasynthesis of women's experiences on VBAC (Vaginal birth after Caesarean section). *BMC Pregnancy and Childbirth, 12*(1), 85.

McDonald, E. A., & Brown, S. J. (2013). Does method of birth make a difference to when women resume sex after childbirth? *BJOG: An International Journal of Obstetrics & Gynaecology, 120*(7), 823-830.

Mohrbacher, N. (2011). The magic number and long-term milk production. *Clinical Lactation, 2*(1), 15-18.

Moran-Peters, J. A., Zauderer, C. R., Goldman, S., Baierlein, J., & Smith, A. E. (2014). A quality improvement project focused on women's perceptions of skin-to-skin contact after cesarean birth. *Nursing for Women's Health, 18*(4), 294-303.

Moore, E. R., Anderson, G. C., Bergman, N., & Dowswell, T. (2012). Early skin-to-skin contact for mothers and their healthy newborn infants. *Cochrane Database of Systematic Reviews, 5,* Published online.

Neville, C. E., McKinley, M. C., Holmes, V. A., Spence, D., & Woodside, J. V. (2014). The effectiveness of weight management interventions in breast-feeding women: A systematic review and critical evaluation. *Birth, 41*(3), 223-236.

Noble, L. M. (2012). Benzodiazepine use safe during lactation. *AAP Grand Rounds, 28*(2), 22-22.

O'Hara, M. W. (2013). *Postpartum depression: Causes and consequences.* Springer-Verlag.

Odom, E. C., Li, R., Scanlon, K. S., Perrine, C. G., & Grummer-Strawn, L. (2013). Reasons for earlier than desired cessation of breastfeeding. *Pediatrics, 131*(3), e726-e732.

Perez, A., Labbok, M. H., & Queenan, J. T. (1992). Clinical study of the lactational amenorrhoea method for family planning. *The Lancet, 339*(8799), 968-970.

Pillitteri, A. (2014). *Maternal & child health nursing, 7ᵗʰ Ed.*. Philadelphia: Lippincott Williams & Wilkins.

Polachek, I. S., Harari, L. H., Baum, M., & Strous, R. D. (2012). Postpartum post-traumatic stress disorder symptoms: The uninvited birth companion. *Israeli Medical Association Journal, 14*(6), 347-353.

Puia, D. (2013). A meta-synthesis of women's experiences of cesarean birth. *MCN: The American Journal of Maternal/Child Nursing, 38*(1), 41-47.

Puryear, L. J. (2007). *Understanding your moods when you're expecting: Emotions mental health and happiness before during and after pregnancy.* New York: Houghton Mifflin Company.

Quinn, T. J., & Carey, G. B. (1999). Does exercise intensity or diet influence lactic acid accumulation in breast milk? *Medicine and Science in Sports and Exercise, 31*, 105-110.

Raymond, N. C., Pratt, R. J., Godecker, A., Harrison, P. A., Kim, H., Kuendig, J., & O'Brien, J. M. (2014). Addressing periatal depression in a group of underserved urban women: A focus group study. *BMC Pregnancy and Childbirth, 14*(1), 336.

Renfrew, M. J., McCormick, F. M., Wade, A., Quinn, B., & Dowswell, T. (2012). Support for healthy breastfeeding mothers with healthy term babies. *Cochrane Database of Systematic Reviews, 5.*

Ricci, S. S., Kyle, T., & Carmen, S. (2013). *Maternity and pediatric nursing*. Philadelphia: Lippincott Williams & Wilkins.

Rice-Simpson, K., & Creehan, P.A. (2014). *Perinatal nursing, 4th Ed.*. Philadelphia: Lippincott Williams and Wilkins.

Sachs, H. C., Frattarelli, D. A., Galinkin, J. L., Green, T. P., Johnson, T., Neville, K. ... Van den Anker, J. (2013). The transfer of drugs and therapeutics into human breast milk: an update on selected topics. *Pediatrics, 132*(3), e796-e809.r

Scharff, K. (2004). *Therapy demystified: An insider's guide to getting the right help (without going broke)*. New York: Marlowe and Company.

Sears, W., Sears, M., Sears, R., & Sears, J. (2013). *The baby book, revised edition: Everything you need to know about your baby from birth to age two*. New York: Little, Brown.

Seetharaman, S., Andel, R., McEvoy, C., Aslan, A. K. D., Finkel, D., & Pedersen, N. L. (2015). Blood glucose, diet-based glycemic load and cognitive aging among dementia-free older adults. *Journals of Gerontology Series A: Biological Sciences and Medical Sciences, 70*(4), 471-479.

Semenic, S. E., Callister, L. C., & Feldman, P. (2004). Giving birth: The voices of Orthodox Jewish women living in Canada. *Journal of Obstetric, Gynecologic, and Neonatal Nursing, 33*(1), 80–87.

Sober, S., & Schreiber, C. A. (2014). Postpartum contraception. *Clinical Obstetrics and Gynecology, 57*(4), 763-776.

Spatz, D. L. (2012), Breastfeeding is the cornerstone of childhood nutrition. *Journal of Obstetric, Gynecologic, & Neonatal Nursing, 41*, 112–113. doi: 10.1111/j.1552-6909.2011.01312.x

Stone, S., Prater, L., & Spencer, R. (2014). Facilitating skin-to-skin contact in the operating room after cesarean birth. *Nursing for Women's Health, 18*(6), 486-499.

Sutton, A.L. (2009). *Pregnancy and birth sourcebook, 3rd. Ed.* Detroit, MI: Omnigraphics Inc.

Taimur, S. D. M., Haq, M. M., Khan, S. R., Kabir, C. S., Rahman, H., Karim, M. R., & Salahuddin, M. (2013). A young lady with acute pulmonary embolism after caesarean section—a case report. *BIRDEM Medical Journal, 3*(2), 116-120.

Urwin, H. J., Miles, E. A., Noakes, P. S., Kremmyda, L. S., Vlachava, M., Diaper, N. D., & Yaqoob, P. (2012). Salmon consumption during pregnancy alters fatty acid composition and secretory IgA concentration in human breast milk. *Journal of Nutrition, 142*(8), 1603-1610.

U.S. Department of Food and Agriculture (USDA): Food and nutrition service. (2014) *Feeding Infants: A guide for use in the child nutrition programs.* http://www.fns.usda.gov/tn/feeding-infants-guide-use-child-nutrition-programs

U.S. Department of Health and Human Services. (2011). *The Surgeon General's Call to Action to Support Breastfeeding.* Retrieved from: http://www.surgeongeneral.gov/library/calls/breastfeeding/ calltoactiontosupportbreastfeeding.pdf

U.S. Department of Health and Human Services. (2013). *Bonding with your baby.* Retrieved from: http://www.childwelfare.gov/pubs/guide2012/bonding.pdf.

Vargas-Martínez, F., Uvnäs-Moberg, K., Petersson, M., Olausson, H. A., & Jiménez-Estrada, I. (2014). Neuropeptides as neuroprotective agents: Oxytocin a forefront developmental player in the mammalian brain. *Progress in Neurobiology, 123*, 37-78.

Venis, J. A., & McCloskey, S. (2007). *Postpartum depression demystified: An essential guide to understanding and overcoming the most common complication after childbirth.* New York: Da Capo Press.

Wainer-Cohen, N., & Estner, L.J. (1983). *Silent knife: Cesarean prevention & vaginal birth after cesarean.* New York: Bergin & Garvey Publishers.

West, D., & Marasco, L. (2009). *Breastfeeding mother's guide to making more milk*. New York: McGraw-Hill.

Williams, K., Donaghue, N., & Kurz, T. (2013). "Giving guilt the flick"? An investigation of mothers' talk about guilt in relation to infant feeding. *Psychology of Women Quarterly, 37*(1), 97-112.

Wirihana, L. A., & Barnard, A. (2012). Women's perceptions of their health-care experience when they choose not to breastfeed. *Women and Birth, 25*(3), 135-141.

Zauderer, C. R. (2008). A case study of postpartum depression and altered maternal newborn attachment. *MCN: The American Journal of Maternal Child Nursing, 33*(3), 173–178.

Zauderer, C. R. (2009). Maternity care for Orthodox Jewish couples: Implications for nurses in the obstetrical setting. *Nursing for Women's Health, 13*(2), 112–120.

Zauderer, C. R. (2009). Postpartum depression: How childbirth educators can help break the silence. *Journal of Perinatal Education, 18*(2), 23–31.

Zauderer, C. R. (2014). PTSD after childbirth: Early detection and treatment. *The Nurse Practitioner, 9*(3), 36-41.

Zauderer, C. R., & Davis, W. (2012). Treating postpartum depression and anxiety naturally. *Holistic Nursing Practice, 26*(4), 203-209.

Zauderer, C. R., & Galea, E. (2010). Breastfeeding and depression: Empowering the new mother. *British Journal of Midwifery, 18*(2), 88–91.

Zuniga, K., & McAuley, E. (2015). Considerations in selection of diet assessment methods for examining the effect of nutrition on cognition. *The Journal of Nutrition, Health, & Aging, 19*(3), 333-340.

Recommended Readings

American College of Obstetricians and Gynecologists (4th Ed.). (2005). *Your pregnancy & birth: Information you can trust from the leading experts in women's health care.* Washington, DC: American College of Obstetricians and Gynecologists.

Audelo, L. (2013). *The virtual breastfeeding culture: Seeking mother-to-mother support in the digital age.* Amarillo, TX: Praeclarus Press.

Behan, E. (2012). *Eat well, lose weight, while breastfeeding: The complete nutrition book for nursing mothers.* New York: Random House.

Bennett, S. S. (2011). *Postpartum depression for dummies.* Edison, NJ: John Wiley & Sons.

Bennett, S., & Indman, P. (2015). *Beyond the blues: Understanding and treating prenatal and postpartum depression & anxiety.* San Francisco, CA: Untreed Reads Publishing.

Brandon, B, & Rupe, H. (2013). *The everything guide to pregnancy nutrition & health: From preconception to post-delivery, all you need to know about pregnancy nutrition, fitness, and diet!* Blue Ash, OH: Adams Media.

Briggs, G. G., & Freeman, R. K., (2014). *Drugs in pregnancy and lactation: A reference guide to fetal and neonatal risk* (10th Ed.). Philadelphia, PA: Wolters Kluwer.

Brott, A. A. (2004). *The new father: A dad's guide to the first year.* New York: Abbeville Press.

Brott, A. A., & Ash, J. (1995). *The expectant father.* New York: Abbeville Press.

Byam-Cook, C. (2012). *Top tips for bottle-feeding.* London: Random House.

Casemore, S. (2013). *Exclusively pumping breast milk: A guide to providing expressed breast milk for your baby.* Napanee, ON , Canada: Gray Lion Publishing.

Cockrell, S., O'Neill, C., & Stone, J. (2007). *Babyproofing your marriage: How to laugh more, argue less, and communicate better as your family grows.* Hebron, NH: Collins Publishing.

Cole, M. (2012). Lactation after perinatal, neonatal, or infant loss. *Clinical Lactation, 3*(3), 94-100.

Connolly, M., & Sullivan, D. (2004). *The essential C-section guide: Pain control, healing at home, getting your body back—And everything else you need to know about a cesarean birth.* New York: Random House.

Finkelstein, B., Finkelstein, M., & Winter, D. (2009). *Delivery from darkness: A Jewish guide to prevention and treatment of postpartum depression.* Jerusalem, Israel: Feldheim.

Flamm, B. L. (1990). *Birth after cesarean: The medical facts.* Upper Saddle River, NJ: Prentice Hall Trade.

Gallagher-Mundy, C. (2004). *Cesarean recovery.* Richmond Hill, ON, Canada: Firefly Books.

Gaskin, I. M. (2008). *Ina May's guide to childbirth: Updated with new material.* New York: Random House.

Greenberg, G., & Hayden, J. (2004). *Be prepared: A practical handbook for new dads.* New York: Simon & Schuster.

Hale, T. W., & Rowe, H. E. (2014). *Medications and mothers' milk, 16th. Ed..* Plano, TX: Hale Publishing.

Hogg, T., & Blau, M. (2011). *Breast-feeding: Top tips from the Baby Whisperer: Includes advice on bottle-feeding.* New York: Simon and Schuster.

HRSA staff. (2008). *The Business Case for Breastfeeding Toolkit: Steps for creating a breastfeeding friendly worksite*. Washington, DC: U.S. Department of Health and Human Services.

Huggins, K. (2015). *The nursing mother's companion: The breastfeeding book mother's trust, from pregnancy through weaning, 7th Ed.*) Boston: Harvard Common Press.

Jones, C. C. (2009). *Eating for pregnancy: The essential nutrition guide and cookbook for today's mothers-to-be*. Cambridge, MA: Da Capo Press.

Jones, R., & Ozer, B.R. (2013). *A dude's guide to babies: The new dad's playbook*. South Portland, ME: Sellers Publishing Inc.

Karp, H. (2008). *The happiest baby on the block: The new way to calm crying and help your newborn baby sleep longer*. New York: Bantam.

Kass-Annese, B., & Danzer, H. C. (2003). *Natural birth control made simple*. Aladmeda, CA: Hunter House.

Kaufmann, E. (1996). *Vaginal Birth After Cesarean: The Smart Woman's Guide to VBAC*. Nashville, TN: Hunter House Publishers.

Kendall-Tackett, K. A. (2005). *The hidden feelings of motherhood: Coping with mothering stress, depression and burnout (2nd. Ed.)*. Amarillo, TX: Hale Publishing.

Klaus, M.H., Kennell, J. H., & Klaus, P. H. (2002). *The doula book: How a trained labor companion can help you have a shorter, easier, and healthier birth*. Boston, MA: Da Capo Press.

Kleiman, K., & Wenzel, A. (2014). *Tokens of affection: Reclaiming your marriage after postpartum depression*. New York: Routledge.

Kleiman, K. (2005). *What am I thinking? Having a baby after postpartum depression*. Bloomington, IN: Xlibris Corporation.

Kleiman, K., & Wenzel, A. (2011). *Dropping the baby and other scary thoughts: Breaking the cycle of unwanted thoughts in motherhood.* New York: Routledge.

Kleiman, K. R. (2001). *The postpartum husband: Practical solutions for living with postpartum depression.* Bloomington, IN: Xlibris Corporation.

Kleiman, K. R., & Raskin, V. D. (2013). *This isn't what I Expected: Overcoming postpartum depression.* New York: Perseus Books Group.

Knight, M. B., & Rosenthal, J. (2010). *Strategies for the C-Section mom: A complete fitness, nutrition, and lifestyle guide.* Avon, MA: Adams Media.

Leach, P. (2013). *Your baby and child.* New York: Knopf.

Lim, R. (2001). *After the baby's birth: A complete guide for postpartum women.* New York: Henry Holt and Company.

Misri, S. (2010). *Shouldn't I be happy?: Emotional problems of pregnant and postpartum women.* New York: Simon and Schuster.

Mohrbacher, N., & Kendall-Tackett, K. (2010). *Breastfeeding made simple: Seven natural laws for nursing mothers, 2nd Ed.* Oakland, CA: New Harbinger Publications.

Mohrbacher, N. (2011). The magic number and long-term milk production. *Clinical Lactation, 2*(1), 15-18.

Murkoff, H. (2005). *What to expect: Eating well when you're expecting.* New York: Workman Publishing.

Nonacs, R. (2006). *A deeper shade of blue: A woman's guide to recognizing and treating depression in her childbearing years.* New York: Simon and Schuster.

Olds, S. W., Marks, L., & Eiger, M. S. (2010). *The complete book of breastfeeding.* New York: Workman Publishing.

Osmond, M., Wilkie, M., & Moore, J. (2008). *Behind the smile: My journey out of postpartum depression*. New York: Grand Central Publishing.

Placksin, S. (2000). *Mothering the new mother: Women's feelings & needs after childbirth: a support and resource guide*. New York: Newmarket Press.

Poulin, S. (2006). *The mother-to-mother postpartum depression support book*. New York: The Berkley Publishing Group.

Puryear, L. J. (2007). *Understanding your moods when you're expecting: Emotions, mental health, and happiness—before, during, and after pregnancy*. Thornwood, New York: Houghton Mifflin Harcourt.

Romm, A. J. (2000). *Naturally healthy babies and children: A common sense guide to herbal remedies, nutrition, and health*. New York: Storey Books.

Romm, A. J. (2002). *Natural health after birth: The complete guide to postpartum wellness*. Rochester, VT: Inner Traditions/Bear & Co.

Rubin, R. (2004). *What if I have a C-section?* New York: Rodale Publishing.

Salt, K. (2002). *A holistic guide to embracing pregnancy, childbirth, and motherhood: Wisdom and advice from a doula*. New York: Basic Books.

Scott, C. C., Hudson, L., MacCorkle, J., & Udy, P. (2007). *Cesarean voices*. Redondo Beach, CA: International Cesarean Awareness Network.

Sears, M., & Sears, W. (2000). *The breastfeeding book*. New York: Little, Brown and Company.

Sears, W., Sears, M., Sears, R., & Sears, J. (2013). *The baby book, Revised Edition: Everything you need to know about your baby from birth to age two*. New York: Little, Brown.

Seip, S. P. (2009). *Momnesia: A humorous guide to surviving your post-baby brain*. Camp Hill, PA: Andrews McMeel Publishing.

Shearer, E. (2012). *Birthing normally after a cesarean or two: A guide for pregnant women exploring practicalities and reasons for VBAC.* Durham, UK: Fresh Heart Publishing.

Shields, B. (2005). *Down came the rain: My journey through postpartum depression.* New York: Hachette Books.

Simpson, B. (2006). *The balanced mom: Raising your kids without losing yourself.* Oakland, CA: New Harbinger Publications.

Solter, A. J. (2001). *The aware baby.* Goleta, CA: Shining Star Press.

Stone, J., & Eddleman, K. (Eds.). (2003). *The pregnancy bible: Your complete guide to pregnancy and early parenthood.* Richmond Hill, ON, Canada: Firefly Books.

Stoppard, M. (2008). *Conception, pregnancy, & birth: The childbirth bible for today's parents.* New York: Penguin Publishing.

Tate, S. (2013). *Into the mouths of babes: A whole foods nutrition guide to feeding your infants and toddlers.* Bloomington, IN: Balboa Press.

Twomey, T. M. (2009). *Understanding postpartum psychosis: A temporary madness.* Westport, CT: Greenwood Publishing Group.

Vadeboncoeur, H. (2011). *Birthing normally after a cesarean or two (American Edition).* Durham, UK: Fresh Heart Publishing.

Venis, J. A., & McCloskey, S. (2007). *Postpartum depression demystified: An essential guide to understanding and overcoming the most common complication after childbirth.* New York: Da Capo Press.

Vieten, C. (2009). *Mindful motherhood: Practical tools for staying sane during pregnancy and your child's first year.* Oakland, CA: New Harbinger Publications.

Wallace, K. (2014). *Reviving your sex life after childbirth: Your guide to pain-free and pleasurable sex after the baby.* Seattle, WA: Kathe Wallace.

Weiner, C. P., & Rope, K. (2013). *The complete guide to medications during pregnancy and breastfeeding: Everything you need to know to make the best choices for you and your baby.* New York: St. Martin's Griffin

West, D., & Marasco, L. (2009). *Breastfeeding mother's guide to making more milk.* New York: McGraw-Hill.

Wider, J. (2008). *The new mom's survival guide: How to reclaim your body, your health, your sanity and your sex life after having a baby.* New York: Bantam.

Wiegartz, P. S., & Gyoerkoe, K. L. (2009). *The pregnancy & postpartum anxiety workbook: Practical skills to help you overcome anxiety, worry, panic attacks, obsessions, and compulsions.* Oakland, CA: New Harbinger Publications.

Wiessinger, D., West, D., & Pitman, T. (2010). *The womanly art of breastfeeding, 8th Ed.* New York: Random House.

Made in the USA
Charleston, SC
24 June 2016